ROBIN FORWARD-WISE is a personal trainer whose love of fitness began with ballet classes at age two. Robin is a certified Pilates instructor whose expertise has been featured in numerous magazines, newspapers, and Pilates instructor manuals. After years of dedicated and intensive study of Pilates, yoga, and ballet, Robin created *Hot Bod Fusion* as a hybrid workout that combines the best of the three disciplines. She is currently a medical student at the University of Arkansas for Medical Sciences.

DAVID WISE is a professional writer with more than fifteen years of experience. He has published hundreds of articles in newspapers and magazines. He is an avid fitness buff who, in addition to *Hot Bod Fusion*, enjoys mountain biking and playing Ultimate. He has a Bachelor of Arts in Journalism and a Master of Science in Mass Communications.

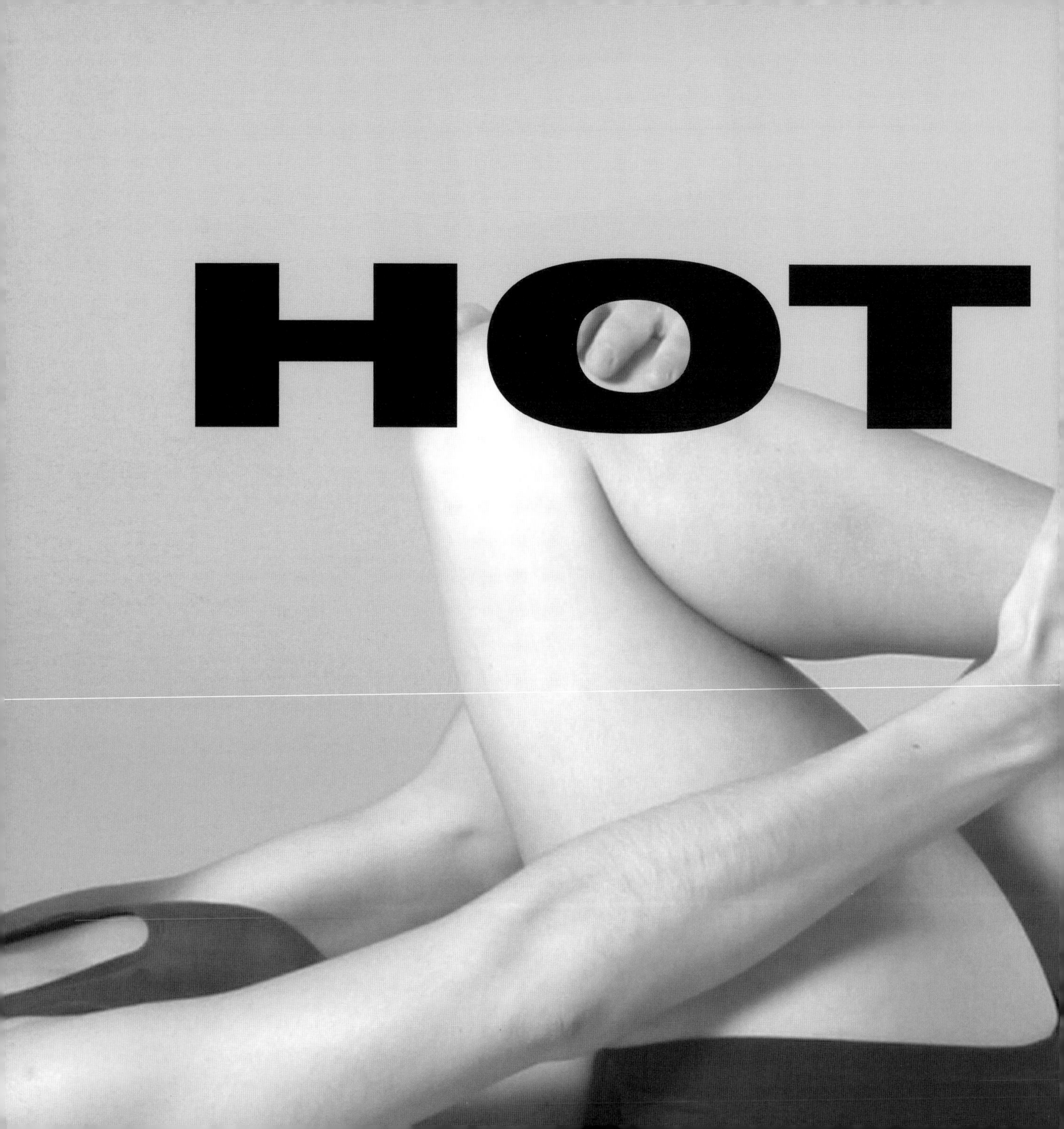
HOT

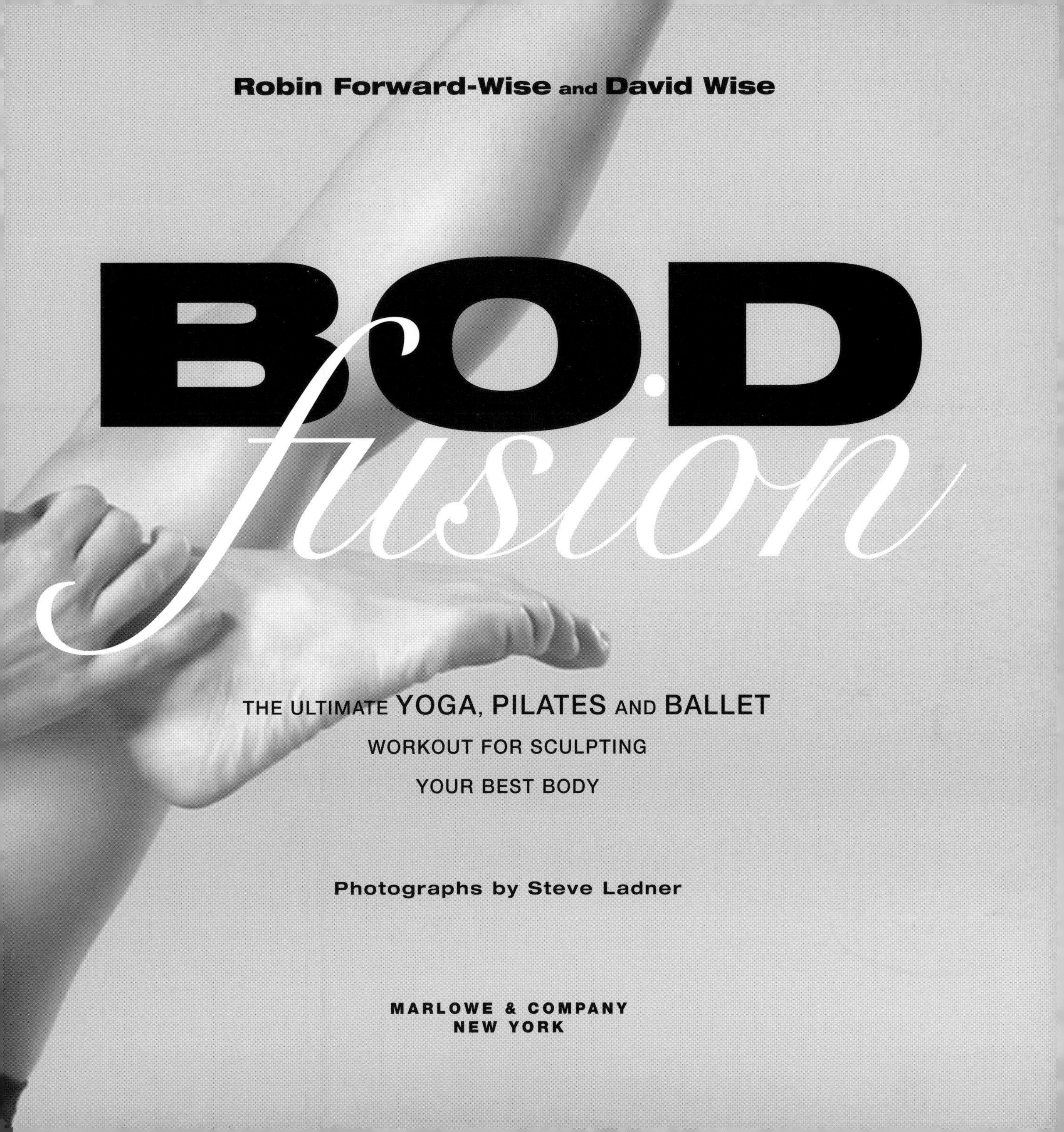

Robin Forward-Wise and David Wise

B.O.D
fusion

THE ULTIMATE YOGA, PILATES AND BALLET

WORKOUT FOR SCULPTING

YOUR BEST BODY

Photographs by Steve Ladner

MARLOWE & COMPANY
NEW YORK

HOT BOD FUSION: *The Ultimate Yoga, Pilates and Ballet Workout for Sculpting Your Best Body*

Copyright © 2004 by Robin Forward-Wise and David Wise
Photographs by Steve Ladner

Published by
Marlowe & Company
An Imprint of Avalon Publishing Group Incorporated
245 West 17th Street • 11th Floor
New York, NY 10011

Library of Congress Cataloging-in-Publication Data is available.

ISBN 1-56924-473-1

9 8 7 6 5 4 3 2 1

Designed by Pauline Neuwirth, Neuwirth and Associates, Inc.

Printed in the United States of America
Distributed by Publishers Group West

To our parents, Robert and Lianne Forward

and George and Hattie Wise

contents

HOT BOD *fusion*

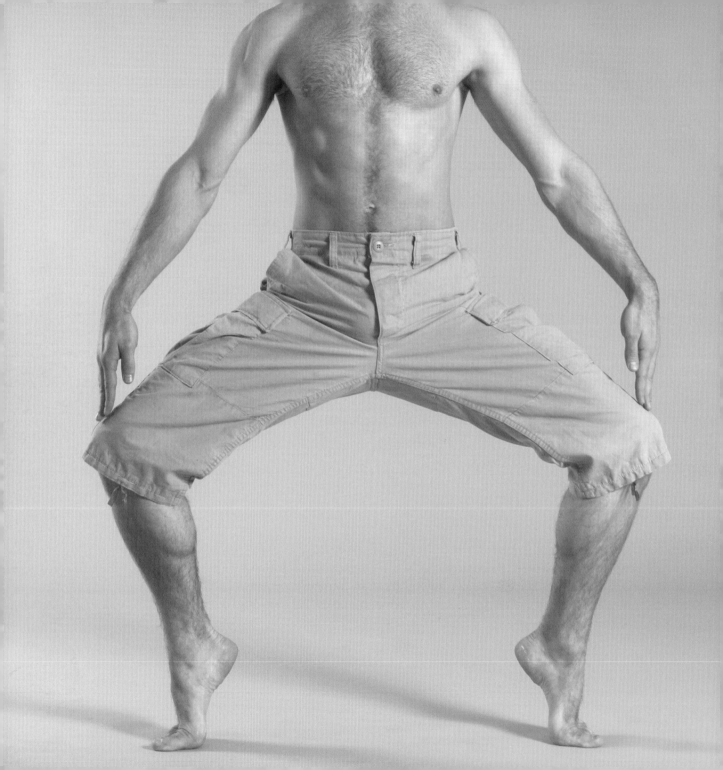

our stories

My **personal journey** into mind-body fitness began when I took my first ballet class at the age of two. I danced all through high school and progressed far enough in my studies to become a student teacher. The lessons I learned in the dance studio became tools that I continue to use in everyday life: I learned to love the human body, to study its functions, and to appreciate the way it moves. Today, I am continuing my ballet education by taking adult classes at a nearby studio.

Classical ballet lessons have shaped many aspects of my life. Ballet even led me to my introduction to Pilates and yoga. Around the time I started college, my sisters (both non-dancers) began touting the transformative benefits of Pilates, claiming that it lifted their spirits and toned their bodies. I was excited to try it, especially when I learned that Pilates had a history of being popular with dancers. After my second year of college, I spent a summer in Los Angeles and finally got my chance to practice Pilates with an instructor. That summer, I also began taking Ashtanga yoga classes (also known as power yoga) in nearby Studio City. I had read a few books on the mind-body benefits of yoga, and I was eager to try Ashtanga in particular because I had heard it was an extremely vigorous style of this age-old discipline. It wasn't long before I was hooked on Pilates, yoga, *and* ballet.

After graduating from college, I longed to find a reputable studio where I could learn more about Pilates and become a certified instructor. I was thrilled to discover that the renowned Stott Pilates main certification center is located in Toronto, where my parents lived and grew up. I spent two summers there taking one-on-one certification classes at the Stott Pilates Studio and received my Pilates Instructor Certification in Pilates matwork and equipment. During this time, I also began taking medical school prerequisites and teaching private and group Pilates classes.

Ballet, Pilates, and yoga have all become an integral part of my lifestyle. As my familiarity with each discipline grew, I was amazed at their similarities. All three disciplines are based on fluid, graceful movements, not jerky repetitions. All three improve concentration and peace of mind. All three increase lean muscle and decrease body fat, keeping you lithe, strong, and flexible. All three necessitate and build a strong core, which decreases shoulder, neck, and back tension.

Making Pilates, yoga, and ballet part of my daily routine was life changing for me, and I wanted to share the benefits of a three-discipline mind-body workout with others. Now that I'm in my first year of medical school, I realize the importance of mind-body fitness and of time-saving workouts as part of a healthy lifestyle even more. That's why I began developing the *Hot Bod Fusion* program. We live in a hectic society, and I wanted to design a fast, full-body workout that would fit into our "on-the-go" schedules.

My familiarity with these three disciplines and how they affected my body and the bodies of my clients helped me to develop the classic exercises featured in this book. I hand picked moves that target specific muscle groups and provide the fastest results: better posture, flatter

INTRODUCTION

abs, stronger arms, leaner legs, and less stress and anxiety. I also chose exercises that would optimally strengthen your core by moving your spine in every direction. I wanted this program to be accessible to everyone, so all of these exercises can be modified or intensified to fit your personal fitness level and each workout combination is only thirty minutes long. That's right— it only takes thirty minutes a day to transform your body and reinvigorate your mind, and if you practice the *Hot Bod Fusion* program consistently, it will positively change your life and your body in just a matter of weeks.

—*Robin Forward-Wise*

I approached fusion workouts from a completely different direction than Robin. Whereas her first love was ballet, my workouts were completely sports-oriented. In fact, when I first met Robin, I was practicing yoga as a way to rehabilitate from injuries I had suffered playing Ultimate, a physically demanding and high-impact sport. I am also an avid mountain biker, and I had found yoga to be an effective tool for stretching my muscles and strengthening my lower back. Due to my competitive nature, however, I was frustrated with my progress because I wasn't the most coordinated or limber person in my class. Robin encouraged me to stick with it and helped me to realize that yoga is not a competitive sport.

She also suggested that I add Pilates to my routine. I was only vaguely familiar with Pilates at the time and I was skeptical at first, but Robin was enthusiastic about its rehabilitative and core-strengthening attributes. I did some research, and after finding quite a few articles about professional athletes using Pilates as part of their training, I decided to give it a try. After just a few sessions, I was hooked. A lot of the movements were similar to yoga, but the workout seemed much more intense and focused. I was also attracted to the mind-body aspect of Pilates, something I had already begun to develop through yoga.

Pretty soon, I was a strong advocate for both yoga and Pilates. When Robin came to me with the idea of collaborating on *Hot Bod Fusion*, I was excited to try the third part of the system, ballet. I'm not a dancer, so I wasn't sure what ballet would add to my workout. But I have never been afraid to try something new, and I was amazed to find that ballet forced me to use muscles I had never challenged before.

Incorporating three different disciplines into one fusion workout has done wonders for my body and my enthusiasm. With all the possible exercise combinations, I get the full-body workout I need, and I never get bored. I encourage you to try *Hot Bod Fusion* for yourself. Whether you're an accomplished athlete or a determined beginner, this program will reshape your body and revitalize your workout routine.

—*David Wise*

INTRODUCTION

what is *hot bod fusion?*

*H*ot Bod Fusion is an extremely effective, easy-to-use workout guide that combines Pilates, ballet, and yoga for a unique hybrid workout that targets the total body. After years of studying, teaching, and performing exercises from these three fitness disciplines, we hand-picked the most effective moves from each and created a workout program that allows you to mix and match sections so you have sixteen different thirty-minute workouts to choose from. We have seen and felt the difference that these exercises can make in only minutes a day. We want you to benefit from our discovery.

THE BEST OF THE BEST

You're probably already aware that Pilates, yoga, and ballet are all great ways to tone your body, boost your energy, improve your balance, heighten your flexibility, relax your mind, increase your stamina, and alleviate stress and tension, but here's a little background on these three amazing ways to keep fit.

PILATES

Pilates integrates muscle control, stretching, and core strengthening into your workout to produce a lean physique through proper alignment and balance. It targets the "core" of your body, which consists of your abs, lower back, and glutes.

Pilates may seem like a relatively new fitness craze, but this mind-body discipline was actually created in the 1920s by German athlete/gymnast Joseph Pilates (1880–1967).

Joseph Pilates suffered from several ailments as a child, most notably asthma, rickets, and rheumatic fever. Determined to overcome his physical liabilities, he studied both Eastern and Western forms of exercise, including yoga, Zen, and ancient Greek and Roman regimens. He used this knowledge to design his own method of conditioning.

Originally called Contrology, Pilates incorporates six principles:

- **Concentration**—You must be conscious of the exercises and focus on what is correct or incorrect.
- **Control**—You can't just throw your body around; every movement must be calculated.
- **Centering**—You need to work both sides of your body evenly.
- **Flow**—Imagine your workout as a dance where every movement flows into the next.
- **Precision**—Exercising correctly is more important than repetition, and you must work on perfecting the details.
- **Breath**—You need to learn to breathe deeply and rhythmically so you can use it as a tool to enhance your performance.

This structure demands mental focus. The routines and breathing techniques of Pilates require a concentration that keeps your mind in tune with your body. As you proceed through the exercises, you will learn to develop and increase your awareness of your body and how it moves.

Pilates combines stretching and strengthening of the deep abdominal and back muscles. This in turn promotes proper posture and trunk stability that combine to build strong, toned bodies. Pilates works specific muscles by contracting, holding, and then releasing them. The movements begin in the abdomen and focus on controlling your stomach muscles. In Pilates, you should always think of pulling your navel in toward your spine. That is how you train your stomach to be flat.

When Joseph Pilates first introduced his non-impact program in New York, it was a huge hit among professional dancers for developing strength and endurance while simultaneously building long, even muscle tone. And while dancers have used Pilates for years, non-dancers also rave about the long, lean muscles that the exercises give them.

Robin trained using the Stott Pilates method that was developed by former professional dancer Moira Stott-Merrithew. The Stott method is a contemporary and more anatomically-based form of the original method developed by Joseph Pilates. In particular, the Stott method incorporates modern exercise principles concerning spinal rehabilitation. While Joseph Pilates' original method promoted a flat back, the Stott method restores the natural curve of the spine.

YOGA

Yoga has been around for five thousand years or more. Because of its origins in India and its focus on meditation, many Westerners harbor a misperception that yoga is a religion. It is not. It is simply a way of integrating your body, mind, and spirit to achieve a life balance.

Traditionally defined as a balance of mind and body, yoga promotes a mental and spiritual state of well-being in your innermost self. You achieve this through a slow and steady series of poses called *asanas* that require strength, balance, focus, and flexibility.

Some of the benefits of yoga include stress reduction, improved circulation (flow of blood to and from the heart), increased flexibility and strength, and enhanced concentration.

We chose yoga for the *Hot Bod Fusion* program because it can give you a powerful workout. Yoga poses increase upper-body strength by targeting muscles in the arms, chest, shoulders, and back. Yoga stretches your muscles and can give you a decent cardio workout as well.

The gentle stretching, twisting, and bending movements also promote flexibility in your joints and muscles and improve circulation.

Yoga styles have merged over the years, and new styles have developed. There are now a multitude of different types of yoga to choose from, everything from traditional, spiritual, and meditational yoga to modern routines that demand more energy and physical fitness. There are also any number of hybrids that combine several styles.

Robin originally learned and trained in Ashtanga yoga (also known as power yoga), which is one of the most physically demanding styles. For *Hot Bod Fusion*, however, we chose to use Hatha yoga. This is a category of yoga in which several styles are grouped into a method that is accessible to people of all fitness and experience levels.

BALLET

Although some archaeologists have traced a form of dancing back to agricultural societies five thousand to ten thousand years ago, we can safely assume that humans were dancing long before that. And while we can only speculate about the ritualistic or ceremonial nature of these dances, we can be sure of one thing: dancing is part of our human nature. Just watch how naturally it comes to young children.

The origins of dance may predate recorded history, but dancing as a social activity and a form of entertainment is relatively new. Classical ballet as we know it is based on the traditional techniques from the French ballet of the seventeenth and eighteenth centuries, and the Italian school of the nineteenth century. *Le Ballet Comique de la Reine* (The Queen's Ballet Comedy), the first ballet for which a complete score survived, was performed in Paris in 1581. The court ballet reached its peak during the reign of Louis XIV (1643–1715), whose title, the Sun King, was derived from a role he danced in a ballet.

We chose ballet for *Hot Bod Fusion* because of its ability to create a long, lean, and elegant body. Like the other disciplines in this book, ballet is rooted in the body's core. Dancing requires a very strong abdominal and back area. You have to be aware of your midsection because every movement demands exact precision and control.

Ballet also promotes stamina, strength, and endurance. Dancers are athletes. You may say that you are neither a dancer nor an athlete. Well, fear not. The ballet moves that we chose for this book are accessible to all levels, even to people who have never danced before in their lives. When creating *Hot Bod Fusion*, one of our main goals was to design a program that provides the benefits of ballet in a way that is not intimidating to those who have never danced.

Ballet dancers develop a heightened sense of their bodies. This is apparent not only when they are performing, but also in their daily lives. There is a visible poise and grace to ballet dancers that distinguishes them from others. If you know any dancers, you have probably noticed how they walk into a room with a natural confidence. The way that you sit, stand, or walk can have a huge impact on the way you look and feel and how other people perceive you. The ballet portion of *Hot Bod Fusion* will not turn you into a professional dancer, but you will reap some of the same benefits that dancers enjoy.

the benefits of
a fusion workout

*I*t's easy to start an exercise regimen; the hard part is sticking with it. Many people soon become bored with the repetition and give up because they no longer feel motivated. It's been said that variety is the spice of life, and exercise is no different.

If you are like us, you are always looking for new ways to have fun when you work out. That's one of the reasons we were first attracted to fusion programs. After years of fitness training, we found that by combining several disciplines into one program we could add a much-needed variety to keep us energized, challenged, and excited about working out.

Our favorite discovery, however, was that fusion workouts boosted our overall fitness level. Whereas traditional workouts, like weight training, are based on targeting individual muscles, a fusion program conditions the muscles in your entire body.

Fusion workouts help you develop strength, endurance, flexibility, proper breathing technique, and improved posture—all with one program. You will become more aware of your body and how it moves. Your confidence will rise. You will begin to carry yourself with more grace and elegance. You will walk into a room with more self-assurance than ever before.

The three *Hot Bod Fusion* disciplines provide you a triple dose of core training, flexibility, and poise. In many ways, these three disciplines are very similar. Each emphasizes mind-body awareness, each emphasizes controlled breathing, and each encourages long, smooth movements. Also, there are no mindless routines. Everything has a purpose and requires complete focus.

CORE TRAINING

Core training means you are working to strengthen the muscles of your entire torso area, including your abs, lower back, and glutes.

Training your core is the most important thing you can do to maintain long-term fitness. Athletes have long known that there is a connection between a strong abdomen and overall fitness. A well-conditioned center is the basis for a strong body. Rock-solid abs are not only pleasing to the eye, they also support the rest of the body.

Traditionally, people have relied on crunches to flatten their abs, but today we know that it makes more sense to train your entire core. Core training works all of the abdominal groups, including the deep muscles that lie near the spinal column. These internal muscles are what shape your waistline. Strengthening your core also gives you better overall control of your entire body, which will help you develop better balance and improved posture. You will stand taller, walk with poise, and project a confident appearance.

CENTERING

Centering is a mind/body technique that yoga practitioners, ballet dancers, Pilates enthusiasts, and other athletes use to maintain a focus on the center of their bodies.

Some people see it as a spiritual self-awareness; others view it in purely physical terms. However you approach it, centering is a crucial element in the *Hot Bod Fusion* workout. You will want to center yourself before each exercise.

Centering is not a difficult concept to master. It is simply a way of focusing your mind on your body. The first step is to close your eyes and pay attention to your breath moving in and out of your lungs. Pay attention to your heartbeat. Now gather all your thought into what you feel is the center of your body. The location is up to you. You can try several different places until you find one where you feel you the most balanced and comfortable. That is the place from which you should begin each exercise.

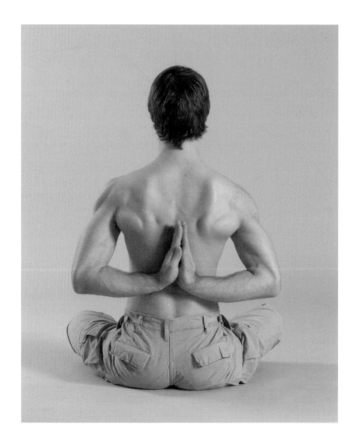

INTRODUCTION

how to use this book

Hot Bod Fusion is broken down into four phases:

Phase One	Five-Minute Beginning Movements	(Chapter 2)
Phase Two	Ten-Minute Total-Body Targeters	(Pick one from Chapters 3, 4, 5, 6)
Phase Three	Ten-Minute Total-Body Targeters	(Pick one from Chapters 7, 8, 9, 10)
Phase Four	Five-Minute Final Stretch	(Chapter 11)

For each workout, you will begin with the warm-up in Phase One and finish with the cool-down in Phase Four. In between, you will pick one chapter from Phase Two and one chapter from Phase Three. For example, on one day your routine might include Chapters 2, 4, 9, 11. On another day, you can switch it up to include Chapters 2, 6, 7, 11.

The four phases add up to only thirty minutes—a perfect fit for even the busiest of schedules.

Since you can mix and match the exercises in Phase Two and Phase Three any way you like, you have access to sixteen different workout combinations that will keep you motivated with fresh possibilities. No matter what combination you choose, the benefits are the same. Each session will yield an effective workout.

We suggest you perform the workout three times a week, alternating days as you go. On the alternate days, you should perform at least twenty minutes of some form of cardiovascular activity, such as walking, running, aerobics, swimming, or tennis.

We have provided some handy progress charts in Chapter 12 to help you keep on track. And if you're not ready to create your own workout yet, you'll also find two sample sequence guides that you can follow.

about the exercises

*T*here are easy-to-follow written directions for every exercise, which are accompanied by quick-reference photos of each movement. The photos will be especially beneficial in helping you achieve proper body alignment.

TIP FROM YOUR PERSONAL TRAINER

Along the way you will find anatomy hints called "Tip from Your Personal Trainer." These are intended to optimize your results and to point out common mistakes to avoid as you work out. These hints are like having a personal trainer in the room with you, guiding you through the details behind the technique, including breathing and alignment principles. Remember, good technique fosters faster results.

EXERCISE INSIGHTS AND ANATOMY VISUALS

At the beginning of each exercise, we'll tell you what body part or parts it targets. This will help you focus your mind and get the most out of your workout. Remember, the purpose of a mind-body workout is to concentrate on using your body efficiently. Knowing which exercises target which muscles will also help you when you are ready to customize your workout to your particular fitness needs and desires.

INTRODUCTION

MODIFIERS AND INTENSIFIERS

It is important to work at a level that is comfortable for you and never to force the exercise. With this in mind, we've included ways to make the exercises easier or harder, depending on your personal level of fitness. In other words, you can adjust the workout to your comfort level. If you feel certain exercises are too hard, the modifiers will provide alternative solutions. On the other hand, if the exercise does not seem to be providing enough of a challenge, the intensifiers will allow you to take the move to a higher level of difficulty. These modifiers and intensifiers will enable you to work out at your own pace. Remember—quality is more important than quantity.

OPTIONAL EXERCISES

Hot Bod Fusion includes two optional Pilates chapters (4 and 8) devoted to exercises that use an inexpensive piece of equipment known as an "exercise circle." The exercise circle incorporates resistance training into basic Pilates moves to provide a new intensity to the Pilates portion of your workout. The exercise circle is readily available at many discount retailers, fitness stores, and on Web sites that sell fitness equipment.

equipment

*T*he *Hot Bod Fusion* program doesn't require much equipment or space, and what you do need is inexpensive and readily available in fitness stores, discount retail stores, and online. You may have some of these items already.

EXERCISE MAT

A quality exercise mat will serve two purposes. First, it will protect your vertebrae from the hard floor or carpet. Second, the sticky surface will provide traction to keep your bare feet from sliding around during the exercises.

EXERCISE CIRCLE (optional)

There are two chapters (4 and 8) in this book that utilize an inexpensive piece of equipment called an exercise circle. The chapters are optional, but you can include them if you want to add a higher level of intensity to the Pilates portion of your workout.

BALLET BARRE

Since most people don't have a ballet barre in their home, we suggest you use a chair back or table for support during the ballet exercises. Alternatively, you could purchase a portable ballet barre.

PILLOW OR BOLSTER (optional)

There are some exercises in this book where we suggest that you use a pillow or bolster for support. You can use it to support your neck or to sit on if you feel discomfort.

CLOTHING

While there are clothing lines made specifically for Pilates, yoga, and ballet, you can probably find a suitable outfit in your closet. Choose comfortable clothes, like lightweight pants and a T-shirt. Although there are many wonderful synthetic, sweat-wicking fabrics on the market that will make an intense exercise session more comfortable, cotton is fine for most workouts. We suggest that you take off your shoes and peel off your socks for this workout. Bare feet will keep you from sliding around by allowing your toes to grip the mat.

WORKOUT SPACE

Find an area that is large enough for you to stretch out the entire length of your body with your arms extended overhead and/or out to your sides. Make sure you can stand up and turn around freely without bumping into anything or feeling crowded.

MIRROR (optional)

Some people like to work out in front of a mirror so they can monitor their progress and make sure their body positioning and alignment are correct. However, others find it intimidating or distracting. If you find it helpful, by all means use one. There is nothing more exciting and encouraging than seeing your body develop like you've always dreamed it would.

tips and cautions

HYDRATION

Drink plenty of fluids before, during, and after your workout. Staying hydrated will keep your body and mind operating at peak performance. Muscle function, reaction time, and aerobic endurance will all be heightened if you keep properly hydrated. Not only that, a well-hydrated body is less prone to side stitches and cramps. You should avoid carbonated and alcoholic beverages before you work out. Caffeine and alcohol dehydrate the body.

When you exercise, we recommended that you replenish your fluids every twenty minutes. Do not wait until you are thirsty. Especially during vigorous exercise, thirst is not always an adequate indicator that your body needs fluid replenishment. By the time you become thirsty, you may already be dehydrated.

DIET

A full stomach is not conducive to an efficient workout. So do not eat thirty to forty-five minutes prior to exercising. Because there are plenty of resources available on proper diet and nutrition, we will not go into great detail on what to eat. Suffice it to say that a consistent diet high in complex carbohydrates, fruits, and grains will give you the nourishment you need to stay energized and refreshed for your workout. And, of course, stay away from fatty foods. A visit to your local bookstore or library will provide you with a wealth of information on the proper diet and nutrition for your fitness lifestyle.

CARDIO

Although some of the exercises in the *Hot Bod Fusion* workout will get your heart pumping, this program is not a cardiovascular workout in and of itself. Therefore, it is important to incorporate some sort of aerobic exercise into your weekly routine. In the sample programs presented in Chapter 12, we have designated certain days as cardio days. Do not neglect this part of your regimen. There are many forms of cardiovascular exercise that are good for you—walking, running, biking, swimming, hiking, climbing, jogging—pick something you enjoy and get that heart rate up!

LIMIT YOUR DISTRACTIONS

All three of the disciplines featured in *Hot Bod Fusion* require you to pay attention to both your body and your mind. This workout is not about mindless repetition. You should strive to be acutely aware of your body and the muscles you are using. Keep the distractions to a minimum. Turn off the TV. Turn on your answering machine. Concentrate fully on each exercise and on the specific muscles you are using. Pretty soon, you will develop an innate sense of how to control your own body for the most effective and efficient results. This is the essence of a mind-body workout.

PHYSICAL REQUIREMENTS AND LIMITATIONS

Check with your physician before beginning any exercise program. Although we designed *Hot Bod Fusion* to be accessible to people of all fitness levels, you should take this book to your doctor and go over the workout with him or her. If you have high blood pressure, if you are on medication, or if you are pregnant, it is absolutely essential that your physician give you the green light for beginning any exercise regimen. There are ways to modify this workout to fit your individual physical needs, but be sure to work this out with your doctor before you begin.

This program is not an exception to the rules of common sense. Even if your doctor has given you permission to perform the *Hot Bod Fusion* workout, do not exercise if you feel pain, dizziness, or when you are sick. Know your own strengths and weaknesses. If you are not comfortable doing a particular exercise, follow the modifications that accompany the exercise or skip it completely.

PREGNANCY

We do not recommend all of the exercises in this book for pregnant women. Check your local bookstore or library for workouts designed specifically for pregnancy.

Hot Bod Fusion, however, is perfect for both pre- and post-pregnancy body firming. Pilates, yoga, and ballet are all known for their effectiveness in strengthening the muscles that support a growing baby, and the gentle, low-impact nature of *Hot Bod*'s exercises make it an ideal program for women looking to regain their pre-pregnancy bodies after giving birth. Just be sure to get your doctor's approval before starting the program.

Robin followed the *Hot Bod Fusion* program before she became pregnant, switched to a hybrid pregnancy workout during her pregnancy, and then used the *Hot Bod Fusion* program to get back in shape after the birth of her baby girl. *Hot Bod Fusion* will get you in shape before your pregnancy, inspire you to stay fit during your pregnancy, and give you a solid and achievable plan for getting back the body you had before the baby.

HOT BOD

fusion

THE BASICS:
BREATHING AND BODY ALIGNMENT

ILATES, BALLET, AND YOGA all require that you are aware of your breathing and body alignment during your workout. Focusing on your breathing will encourage you to think about what your body is doing at that moment. Because you will be more in tune with your body (and less in tune with the distractions around you, such as TV, music, or other people talking), you are more likely to exercise correctly, which will increase your results.

Breathing is something you do naturally and automatically all day long. You probably don't give it much thought. However, because proper breathing is such an integral part of all three of the disciplines used in this book, you will need to be aware of how you are breathing in order to get the most out of your workout. Here are just a few reasons why it is so important to develop a strong and deep breathing technique.

Proper breathing:
- oxygenates your blood
- increases circulation
- releases tension, especially in your neck and back
- focuses your mind, allowing you to concentrate on your movements.

As you undoubtedly already know, a breath involves two actions: inhaling and exhaling. As elementary as that sounds, knowing what happens to your body when you inhale and exhale will enhance your mind-body experience, and your workout will rise to a whole new level of effectiveness.

Your blood is made up of oxygen, and correct breathing allows the oxygen to nourish your body. Oxygen-rich blood is vital to good health. Sending fresh oxygen to your muscles relieves tension and stress. Supplying your brain with an ample supply of oxygen will increase your concentration. Without enough oxygen, the body becomes fatigued. Deep breathing increases the level of oxygen in your body, which will make you more energetic and improve your stamina.

Deep breathing also facilitates the release of unwanted chemicals related to stress and fatigue. When you exhale, you release waste carbon dioxide from the blood. Exhaling stale air and noxious gases from the depths of your lungs and replacing it with fresh air will revitalize your system. This will keep you more energetic and boost your endurance during you workout.

Controlling the way you breathe is fundamental to an effective workout. The rhythm of your breathing and your motions are linked together. For many of the exercises in this book, we suggest the correct time to inhale and exhale. For example, when you inhale, oxygen travels to your lungs and there is a natural lifting of your ribs. This is why we often pair an inhale with the preparation movement. Likewise, when you exhale, your ribs drop and your abs tighten, enabling you to exert more power during movement. When the timing is not indicated, you should breathe normally and concentrate on the rhythm of your breathing.

Here are a few tips to keep in mind as you perform the breathing exercises that follow, as well as the exercises throughout the book:

HOT BOD FUSION

- Use full inhalations and full exhalations for a thorough oxygenation of the blood.
- Never, under any circumstances, should you stop breathing. Rather, you should concentrate on breathing through every move.
- In general, you will inhale to prepare for a movement, and exhale as you perform the movement. In other words, exhale as you exert effort.

BREATHING EXERCISES TO GET YOU STARTED

This exercise will help you understand how to integrate proper breathing techniques into your movements. Keep the following two points in mind as you perform the practice exercises that follow:

- An inhale is the natural lifting of ribs (also known as *extension*).
- An exhale is the natural contraction of abs (also known as *flexion*).

arm circles

STARTING POSITION

Begin lying on your back. Bend your knees hip-width apart and rest your arms long by your sides, palms down.

1. Inhale and fill your lungs with air, feeling your rib cage fully expand as you reach your arms toward the ceiling and then lower them backwards until they are stretched out over your head. Keep the back of your rib cage from lifting off the mat by tightening your abs and not lifting your arms so far overhead that you cannot maintain contact with the mat.

2. Now exhale and close your rib cage as you circle your arms out and around to your side and return to Starting Position.

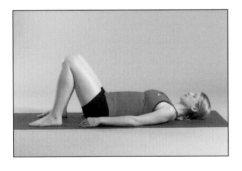 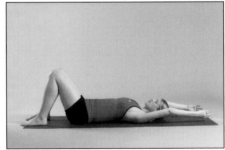

Repeat 3 times.

ab isolation #1—coughing exercise

STARTING POSITION

Begin lying on your back. Bend your knees hip-width apart and rest your arms long by your sides, palms down.

1. Place your fingertips just inside your hipbones and inhale.

2. Now exhale with a cough. You will feel your transversus abdominus tighten as air is released. This is a band of muscle that supports your core like a belt. Try to maintain this tightened feeling. It may be difficult at first, but with practice, you will be able to maintain this tightness throughout the *Hot Bod Fusion* workout. This will help stabilize your lumbar (lower) spine and pelvis while toning your midsection.

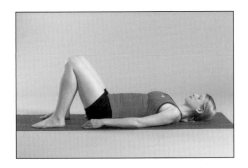 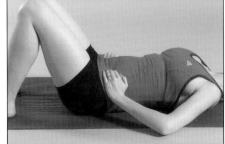

Repeat 3 times.

ab isolation #2—hollow out the abs

STARTING POSITION

Begin lying on your back. Bend your knees hip-width apart and rest your arms long by your sides, palms down.

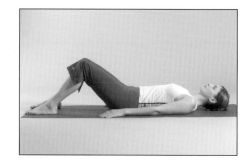

1. Inhale to fill the lower lobes of your lungs, feeling your ribcage expand (this means you should not breathe into your upper chest or your stomach).

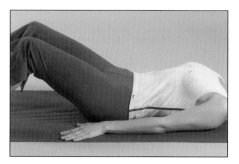

2. Now exhale and pull your naval to your spine to support your back as you hollow out the abdominals. Think of it as "scooping" your abs in toward your spine.

Repeat 3 times.

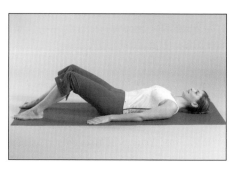

spinal placement for pilates moves

Here are the three main spinal positions that you will use in the Pilates sections:

- **NATURAL POSITION:** This means you are to hold the natural curve of your spine. There will likely be a small space between your lower spine and the mat. You will use this position when your feet are in contact with the mat.

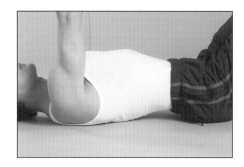

- **IMPRINT POSITION:** This position requires you to lengthen your back muscles against the mat, tighten your abs, and draw your naval down toward your spine. Think of "closing" the space between your spine and the mat. Do not tighten your glutes to find this position. Instead, use your abs, as described in Ab Isolation #2 (page 6), and a slight lift of your tailbone. You will use this position when your feet are not in contact with the mat.

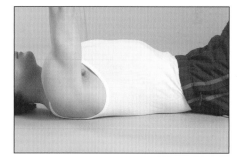

- **C-CURVE POSITION:** Just as it sounds, this position occurs when you roll your spine forward until your back is in the shape of a C. Begin sitting, with your feet planted hip-width apart. Pull your naval to your spine, drop your chin, and roll off your sit bones as you round your spine. You will use this position when you are moving to or from a sitting position on the mat and in Rolling Like a Ball (pictured right).

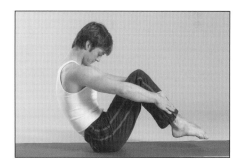

feet placement for ballet

There are actually five basic feet positions in ballet, but for the sake of simplicity, you will only use the first two positions in *Hot Bod Fusion*.

FIRST POSITION

Place your heels together and point your toes outwards to form a V. Keep all your toes on the floor, distribute your weight evenly, and turn your legs out.

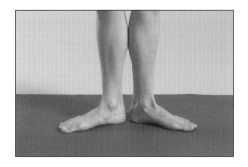

SECOND POSITION

Similar to First Position, but your heels should be apart just wider than your shoulders. As with First Position, point your toes outwards to form a V. Keep all your toes on the floor, distribute your weight evenly, and direct your knees to the side.

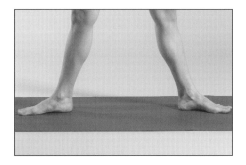

ARM PLACEMENT FOR BALLET

There are multiple arm movements in ballet, but we chose to use a limited number in *Hot Bod Fusion*. Follow along with the pictures in each chapter if you want to add this element to your workout. If not, just leave out the arm movements and place your hands on your hips.

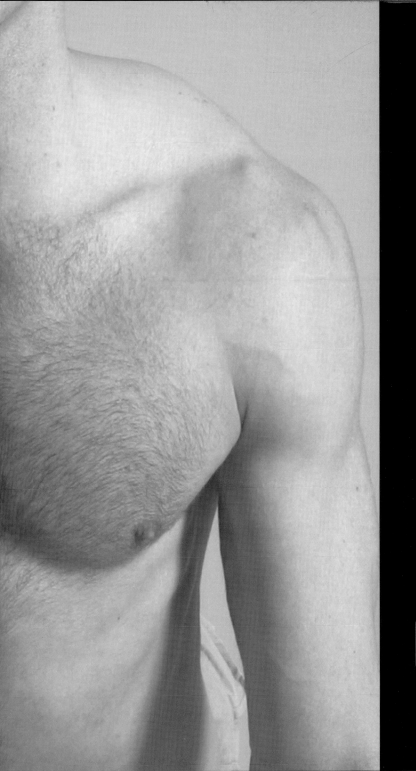

phase one

BEGINNING MOVEMENTS

(Five-minute warm-up)

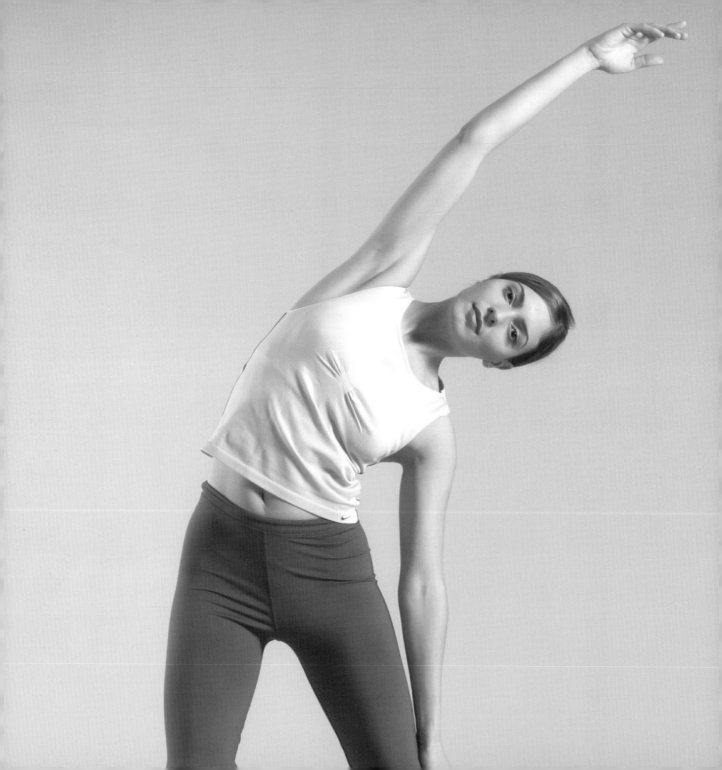

two

THE
WARM-UP

*t*HIS FIVE-MINUTE warm-up melds movements from Pilates, ballet, and yoga. We specifically created these warm-up exercises to prepare your muscles for the *Hot Bod Fusion* workout. It's also a great way to improve your posture and body alignment. Stretching is one of the safest and most natural ways to begin any exercise, and taking time to warm up will help reduce your risk of injury and muscle soreness. So do this warm-up before every exercise session. Your body will thank you for it.

body release

This is a full-body warm-up.

STARTING POSITION

Begin standing with your feet shoulder-width apart.
Relax your shoulders down and back to open up your chest.

1. Inhale and center yourself.

2. Exhale and bend your knees slightly.

3. Inhale and rest your left hand on your left thigh.
   Then raise your right arm up and over your head to the left.

4. Exhale as you drop your head and round your spine,
   lowering your right arm so both hands are resting on your thighs.

5. Inhale again and continue to rest your right hand on
   your right thigh. Then lift your left arm up and over your head to the right.

6. Exhale and straighten your knees, standing tall.

7. Repeat in the opposite direction.

Repeat entire sequence 2 times.

HOT BOD FUSION

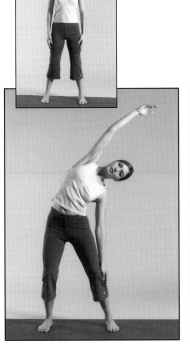

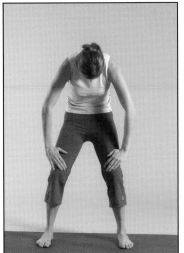

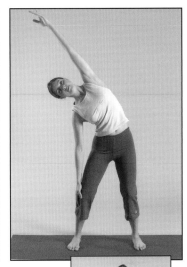

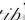 *tip* **from your personal trainer**

Lift up and out through your
hips as you reach your arm
overhead.

THE WARM-UP

13

neck rolls

Use these rolls to release neck tension.

STARTING POSITION

Begin standing with your feet shoulder-width apart.
Relax your shoulders down and back to open up your chest.

1. Inhale and center yourself.

2. Exhale and drop your ear toward one of your shoulders. Slowly drop your chin to your chest and circle your head around to the other side. Pause to hold the stretch.

3. Inhale again and center yourself, then repeat in opposite direction.

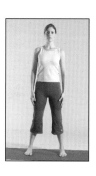 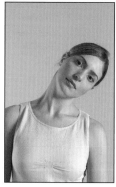 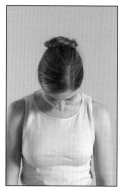 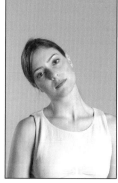 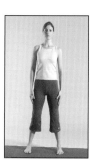

Repeat entire sequence 2 times.

 tip **from your personal trainer**

Keep your shoulders relaxed and down.

cat stretch

This exercise will warm up your spine and release lower back tension.

STARTING POSITION

Begin on hands and knees, with your knees hip-width apart.

1. Inhale and center yourself.

2. Exhale as you drop your tailbone and round your spine one vertebrae at a time, finishing with your head drawn toward your thighs.

3. Inhale again and deepen the stretch by lifting your abs and pulling your naval to your spine.

4. Exhale while you lift your tailbone first, then your head, and finish with a slight extension of the spine.

Repeat 4 times.

tip **from your personal trainer**

If this exercise bothers your knees, place a pillow under your knees.

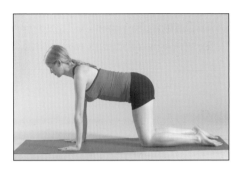

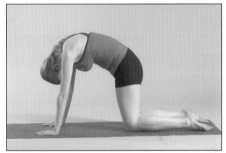

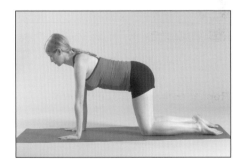

swimming

This exercise focuses on your upper, middle, and lower back, as well as your glutes and your hamstrings. It also improves balance.

STARTING POSITION

Begin on hands and knees, knees hip-width apart.

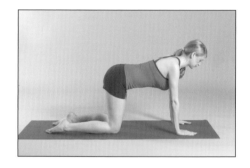

1. Inhale and center yourself.

2. Exhale and pull your naval to your spine as you extend your right arm out in front of you and your left leg straight back. Form one long line from hand to foot.

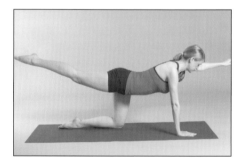

3. Inhale again and keep holding the stretch.

4. Then exhale and lower to Starting Position.

5. Repeat with opposite arm and leg.

Repeat entire sequence 2 times.

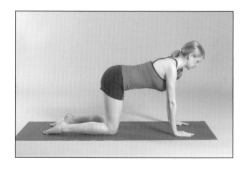

from your personal trainer

Concentrate on reaching your fingers away from your toes and lifting toward the ceiling.

Be careful not to hyperextend your back during this exercise.

TO MODIFY:

Lift your leg and arm one at a time instead of simultaneously.

TO INTENSIFY:

Begin in a push-up position, and stay up on your toes when you extend your arm and leg. Keep your tush low and your abs tight.

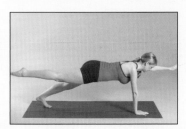

ankle circles/leg circles

Ankle circles will warm up your feet. Leg circles will stretch your leg muscles and strengthen the muscles around your hip joint.

STARTING POSITION

Begin lying on your back, legs stretched out long and arms resting at your sides. Now lift one leg straight up toward the ceiling.

1. Inhale and rotate your ankle in one full circle.

2. Exhale and rotate your ankle in another full circle. Complete 4 full ankle circles in both directions.

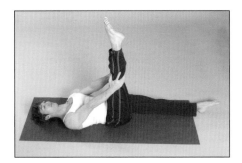 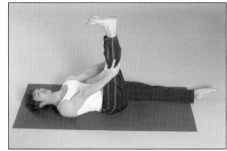

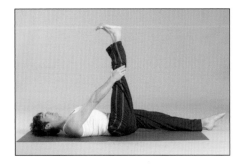 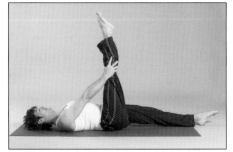

HOT BOD FUSION

3. Inhale and rotate your leg in the hip socket in a bicycle tire-sized circle, sweeping your leg across your body and out to the side.

4. Exhale and rotate your leg in another bicycle tire-sized circle. Complete 4 full leg circles in both directions.

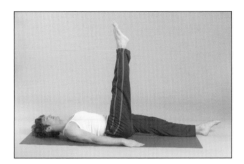 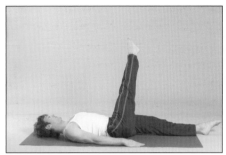

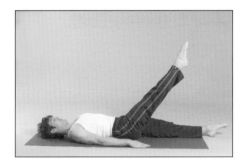 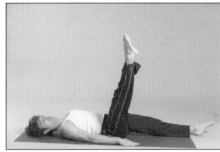

tip **from your personal trainer**

Keep your abs tight. This will stop your hips from moving around on the mat during leg circles.

TO MODIFY:
If you feel pressure on your back or if your hamstrings are tight, try bending your knees.

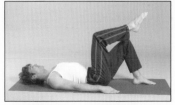

lying torso twist

This move will strengthen your spinal rotators and extensors, while stretching your abs.

STARTING POSITION

Begin lying on your side with your arms out-stretched and stacked at chest height. Keep your hips and knees bent at 90-degree angles and stacked on top of each other.

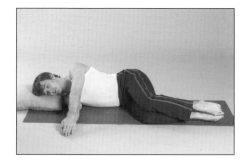

1. Keeping your eyes on your top arm, inhale and reach your top arm toward the ceiling.

2. Exhale and continue to open your arm to your other side. Hold the stretch for two breaths.

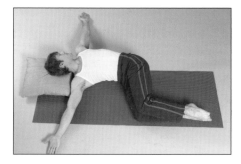

3. Inhale and reach your arm back toward the ceiling.

4. Exhale and return to Starting Position.

Repeat 3 times on both sides.

tip **from your personal trainer**

If your neck placement is uncomfortable, place a pillow under your head.

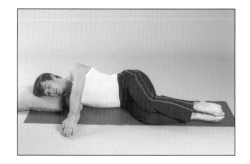

HOT BOD FUSION

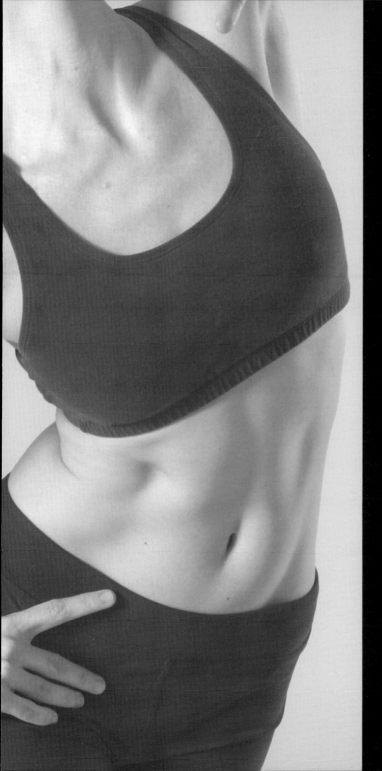

phase two

TOTAL-BODY
TARGETERS
(Ten-minute workout)
Choose either Chapter 3, 4, 5, or 6

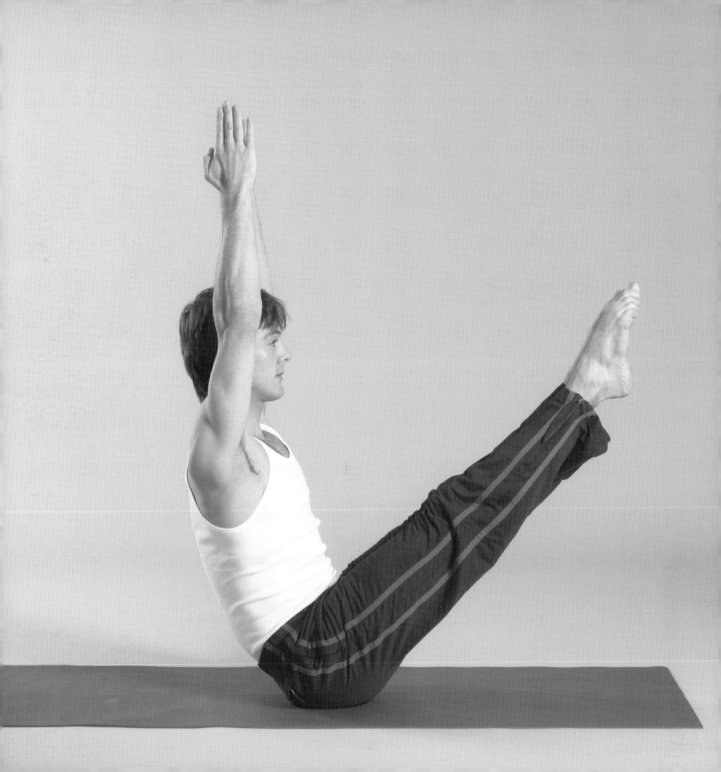

CORE
STRENGTHENERS

PILATES

*T*HIS TEN-MINUTE workout uses Pilates movements to tone the trunk of your body, including your back and abdominals. In Pilates, good form is everything, so concentrate on keeping your movements slow and controlled as you perform these exercises.

the hundred

Use this classic Pilates exercise to get your blood flowing. It also focuses on your abs and the muscles in your arms and shoulders.

STARTING POSITION

Lie on your back with your arms to your sides. Imprint your spine so your whole spine meets the floor. (See page 7 for a refresher on the imprint position for the spine.) Lift your legs and bend your knees to your chest at a 90-degree angle.

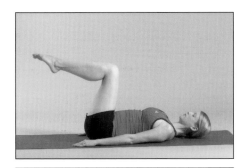

1. Inhale and center yourself. Nod your chin toward your chest so you are looking at your belly button.

2. Simultaneously, raise your legs to a 75- to 90-degree angle. Exhale and using your abs, flex your spine and bring your arms a few inches off the mat.

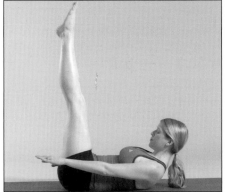

3. Pump your arms up and down in tandem with 5 short inhalations.

4. Keep pumping your arms up and down in tandem with 5 short exhalations.

5. Repeat Steps 3 and 4 a toatl of 10 times, or 100 breaths.

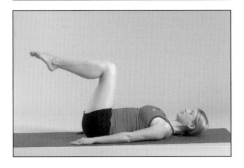

6. Hold your position for one full inhalation, then exhale and roll your upper body down and place your feet back on the mat one at a time. Return your spine to neutral position.

Repeat 10 times.

tip

from your personal trainer

➤ Keep your arms in rhythm with each other and do not bend your wrists. Imagine you are pushing against springs.

➤ If your neck starts to hurt, continue The Hundred with your head resting on the mat.

TO MODIFY:
Bend your knees to 90 degrees in the air. Or you may keep your feet on the floor with your knees bent.

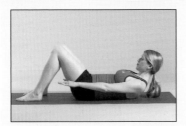

TO INTENSIFY:
Lower your legs closer to the floor, but only so far as you can maintain an imprinted spinal position.

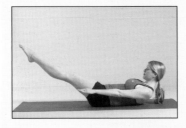

roll up

This move strengthens your abs, and stretches your lower back and hamstrings.

STARTING POSITION

Lie on your back with your spine imprinted. Stretch your arms overhead and hold them about three inches above the mat. Squeeze your outstretched legs together and flex your feet.

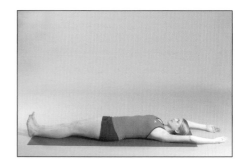

1. Inhale and nod your chin toward your chest and reach your arms to the ceiling.

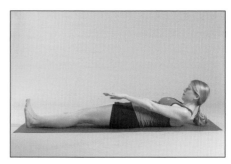

2. Exhale and begin curling your body off the mat one vertebra at a time. Continue the movement as you reach for your toes, rolling your spine into a C-curve.

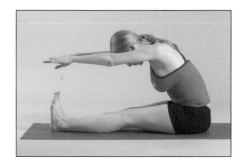

3. Inhale and begin to roll back down toward the mat.

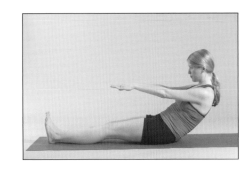

4. Exhale and continue to roll down to the mat one vertebra at a time. Return your arms overhead.

Repeat 6 times.

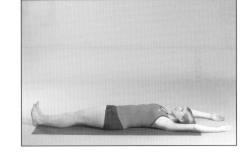

tip **from your personal trainer**

➤ Draw your abdominals in as you round over.
➤ Slide your shoulders away from your ears as you roll down.

TO MODIFY:
Bend your knees.

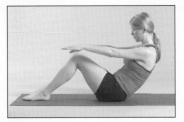

roll over

This exercise targets your abs.

STARTING POSITION

Lie on your back with your spine imprinted. Rest your arms at your sides, palms down. Hold your legs together and reach them up at a 90-degree angle.

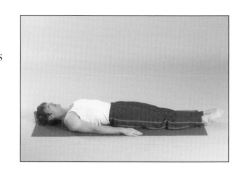

1. Inhale while you contract your abs, keeping your legs extended. Use your abs to lift your tailbone and start to bring your legs overhead.

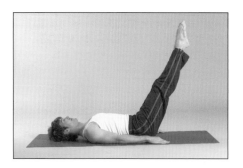

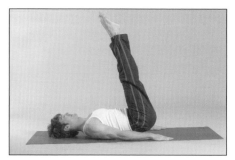

2. Exhale as you roll back on your shoulders and bring your legs all the way over your head until your toes are touching the floor. Avoid rolling onto your neck.

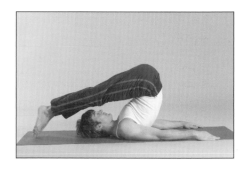

3. Inhale and lift your legs until they are parallel with the floor. Now open your legs to shoulder width.

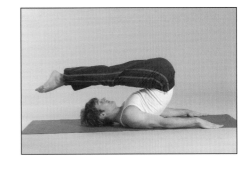

4. Roll your spine back down onto the mat as you exhale and slowly close your legs as you return them to their original 90-degree angle.

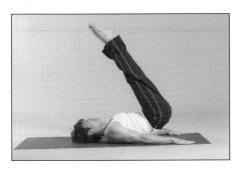
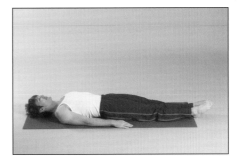

Repeat 10 times.

tip

from your personal trainer

➤ If you have a bad neck, skip this exercise or perform the modified version below.
➤ Remember to keep your arms and palms resting on the floor.
➤ Do not throw your legs over your head. A slow, steady motion is the key to rolling along the center of your spine.

TO MODIFY:
Do not roll back on your shoulders. Roll your tailbone just off the mat and focus on using your lower abs.

CORE STRENGTHENERS ▬

rolling like a ball

This exercise massages your back and builds abdominal strength.

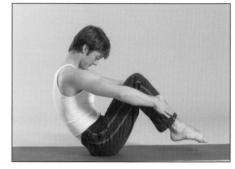

STARTING POSITION

Sit with your legs together, knees bent. Form yourself into a ball by curving your spine and placing your hands on your shins. Roll back off your sit bones, lift your feet just off the mat, and balance.

1. Inhale and roll back onto the mat, maintaining the C-curve of your spine and the contraction of your abs.

2. Exhale and roll back up without changing the ball shape of your body.

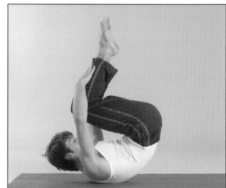

Repeat 10 times.

 tip

from your personal trainer

➤ Roll down the center of your spine.
➤ Be sure not to roll back on your neck.
➤ Do not use your legs for momentum. Keep yourself rolled up into a ball and let your abs do the work.

TO MODIFY:

Skip the roll and hold your balance in Starting Position for 5 breaths.

HOT BOD FUSION

saw

Use this exercise to stretch your hamstrings and lower back.

STARTING POSITION

Begin sitting tall, with your legs stretched out in front of you at shoulder width. Flex your feet and extend your arms straight out to your sides, palms forward.

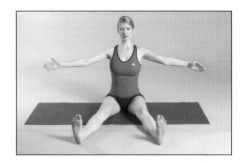

1. Inhale and twist at your waist until one arm is reaching forward and the other is stretched out behind you.

2. Roll from your head down and reach your front hand toward your little toe as you exhale. Reach your back arm in the opposite direction.

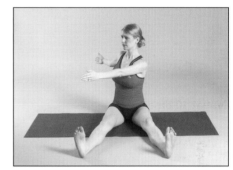

3. Inhale as you tighten your abs and roll up through your spine.

4. Exhale as you rotate back to center.

Repeat 3 times in each direction.

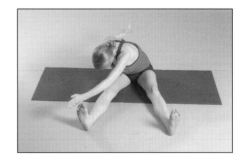

tip **from your personal trainer**

Do not move your hips or legs. Your buttocks should stay glued to the mat.

TO MODIFY:
Sit on a pillow to help stay up on your sit bones.

CORE STRENGTHENERS

one-leg stretch

This exercise increases your coordination, tightens your buttocks and abs, and lengthens the muscles in your legs and hips.

STARTING POSITION

Lie on your back with your spine imprinted. Lift your legs, and bend your knees at a 90-degree angle. Rest your arms at your sides, palms down.

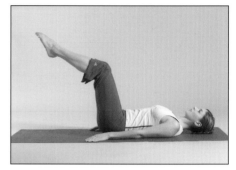

1. Inhale and center yourself while nodding your chin to your chest.

2. Lift your upper body off the mat with an exhale.

3. Inhale again, holding your position.

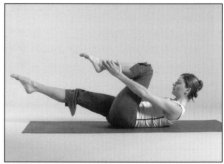

4. Extend your right leg horizontal to the mat as you exhale, moving your left hand to your left ankle and your right hand to your left knee.

5. Inhale and begin to switch your hand and leg positions.

6. Fully extend your left leg horizontal to the mat as you exhale, placing your right hand on your right ankle and your left hand on your right knee.

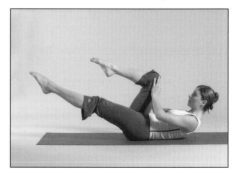

7. Inhale and begin to switch your hand and leg positions.

Repeat 10 times.

tip

from your personal trainer

➤ Just move your arms and legs during this exercise.
  Keep your torso steady.
➤ Concentrate on extending your legs to their maximum.

TO MODIFY:
  Raise your legs higher. Or keep your head on the mat and just
  work your legs.

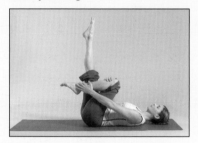

TO INTENSIFY:
  Lower your legs closer to the mat.

one-leg stretch with obliques

This exercise targets the oblique muscles in your waist.

STARTING POSITION

Lie on your back with your spine imprinted. Lift your legs and bend your knees at a 90-degree angle. Place your hands behind your head.

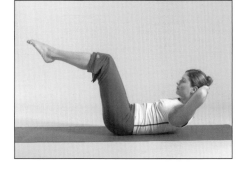

1. Inhale and center yourself.

2. Lift your upper body off the mat with an exhale.

3. Inhale and hold your position.

4. Extend your right leg horizontal to the mat with an exhale while simultaneously rotating your upper body toward your bent left knee.

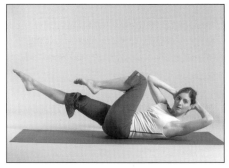

5. Inhale and begin switching your leg positions.

6. Fully extend your left leg as you exhale and rotate your upper body toward your bent right knee.

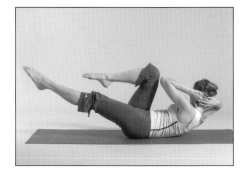

7. Inhale and begin switching your leg positions.

Repeat 10 times.

from your personal trainer

Your elbows should always remain wide. Rotate using your abs, not your arms.

TO MODIFY:
Raise your legs higher. Or keep your feet on the mat and just use your upper body.

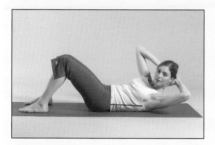

TO INTENSIFY:
Lower your legs closer to the mat.

back extension

This move improves your posture and strengthens your back muscles.

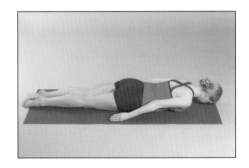

STARTING POSITION

Begin lying flat on your stomach. Rest your arms at your sides, palms in.

1. Inhale as you raise your chest and head off the mat and reach your arms back toward your feet.

2. Exhale and lower yourself back to the mat.

Repeat 6 times.

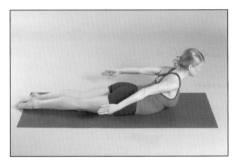

tip **from your personal trainer**

➤ Keep your abs tight to support your lower back.
➤ Keep your legs together and stationary.
➤ Be careful not to overextend your neck.

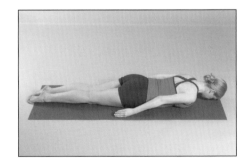

swan dive

This exercise strengthens the muscles in your back, neck, and shoulders.

STARTING POSITION

Begin lying flat on your stomach, legs slightly apart. Place your palms face-down on the mat directly below your shoulders.

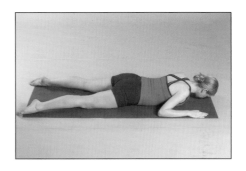

1. Pull your navel toward your spine with an inhale and straighten your arms, arching your back and keeping your head up.

2. Exhale and lengthen into your extension, pull in your abs, and return to the mat.

Repeat 6 times.

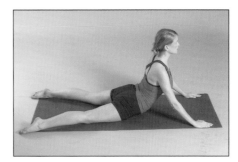

tip

from your personal trainer

➤ Keep your shoulders open and sliding away from your ears.
➤ Keep your elbows down and close to your body.

TO INTENSIFY (unless you have back problems):
As you exhale to return to the mat with your upper body, lift your legs off the mat. As you inhale, lower your legs.

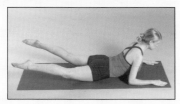

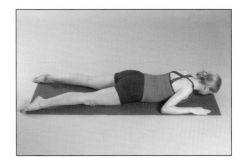

CORE STRENGTHENERS ■

teaser

This classic Pilates exercise is one of the most challenging workouts for your abdominal muscles.

STARTING POSITION

Begin by lying on your back with your spine neutral. Put your feet on the floor, legs together, knees bent. Stretch your arms out behind your head.

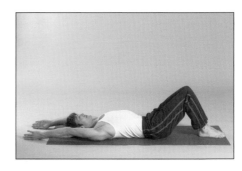

1. Inhale and slowly raise your arms, while dropping your chin to your chest.

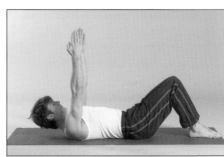

2. Continue your forward arm motion as you exhale and peel your spine off the mat one vertebra at a time until you are sitting upright on your sit bones and your arms are just above your knees.

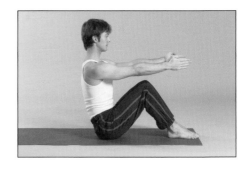

HOT BOD FUSION

3. Inhale and lift your arms toward the ceiling.

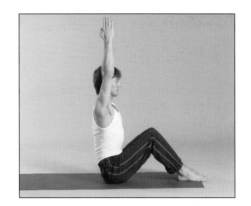

4. Roll your pelvis away from your thighs as you exhale and roll back down onto the mat one vertebra at a time, through the imprint, finishing with your spine neutral and your arms overhead in Starting Position.

Repeat 6 times.

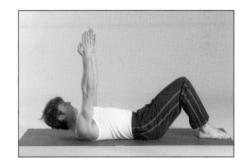

tip **from your personal trainer**

TO INTENSIFY:
Begin and finish with an imprinted spine. Lift your legs up to a 90-degree angle or lower your legs as close to the mat as you can maintain a spinal imprint.

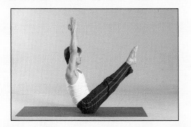

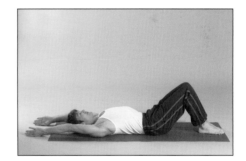

spinal release

This counter-stretch will release and relax your spine.

STARTING POSITION

Begin lying flat on your stomach with your arms stretched out in front of you.

1. Push back with your hands and arms until your hips are resting on your heels. Keep your forehead on the mat and round your spine. Let your arms relax at your sides and breathe normally for several breaths.

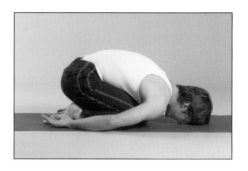

HOT BOD FUSION

four

OPTIONAL CORE STRENGTHENERS
(WITH EXERCISE CIRCLE)

PILATES

HIS TEN-MINUTE section utilizes an exercise circle to add a new level of intensity to your core workout. These movements were chosen specifically to tone your back and abdominals. The key to using an exercise circle is to squeeze it evenly—not in jerky motions or favoring one side of the body.

the hundred

Use this classic Pilates exercise to get your blood flowing. It also focuses on your abs and the muscles in your arms and shoulders.

STARTING POSITION

Lie on your back with your arms to your sides. Imprint your spine so you feel your whole spine meet the floor. Lift your legs and bend your knees to your chest at a 90-degree angle. Hold the circle between your ankles.

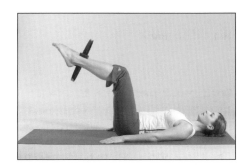

1. Inhale and center yourself. Nod your chin so you're looking at your belly button.

2. Exhale and using your abs, flex your spine as you exhale and bring your arms a few inches off the mat. Simultaneously, raise your legs to a 75 to 90 degree angle..

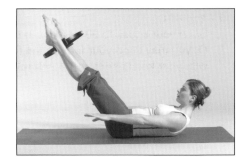

3. Inhale and pump your arms up and down in tandem with 5 short inhalations.

4. Exhale and keep pumping your arms up and down in tandem with 5 short exhalations while squeezing the circle in one smooth motion.

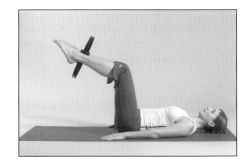

5. Repeat Steps 3 and 4, 10 times, for a total of 100 breaths.

6. Hold your position for one full inhalation. Then exhale and roll your upper body down and place your feet back on the mat one at a time. Return your spine to neutral position.

Repeat 10 times.

tip

from your personal trainer

➤ Keep your arms in rhythm with each other and do not bend your wrists. Imagine you are pushing against springs.
➤ If your neck starts to hurt, continue The Hundred with your head resting on the mat.

TO MODIFY:
Bend your knees to 90 degrees in the air. Or you may keep your feet on the floor with your knees bent, spine neutral.

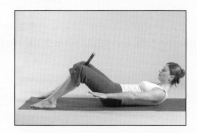

TO INTENSIFY:
Lower your legs closer to the floor only so far as you can maintain an imprinted spinal position.

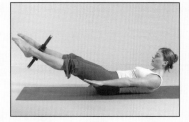

CORE STRENGTHENERS (WITH EXERCISE CIRCLE) ■

roll up

This workout strengthens your abs, and stretches your lower back and hamstrings.

STARTING POSITION

Lie flat on your back, spine neutral, and stretch your arms overhead with the circle between your hands. Squeeze your outstretched legs together and flex your feet.

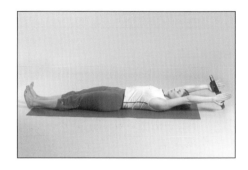

1. Inhale and nod your chin toward your chest, reaching your arms toward the ceiling.

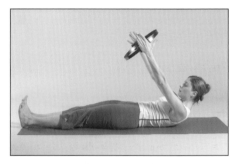

2. Squeeze the circle as you exhale and begin curling your body off the mat one vertebra at a time. Continue the movement as you reach for your toes, rolling your spine into a C-curve.

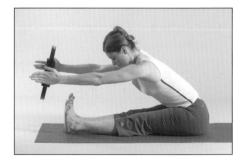

44

3. Inhale and slowly release the tension on the circle as you begin to roll back down toward the mat.

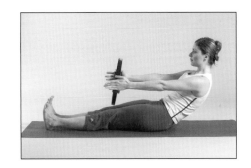

4. Exhale and squeeze the circle as you continue to roll down to the mat one vertebra at a time. Return your arms overhead and release the tension on the circle.

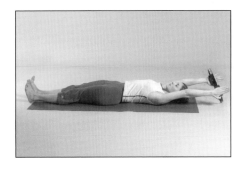

Repeat 6 times.

tip

from your personal trainer

➤ Draw your abdominals in as you curl your body over.
➤ Slide your shoulders away from your ears as you roll down.
➤ Roll your spine through the imprint on the way up and down.

TO MODIFY:
Bend your knees slightly.

CORE STRENGTHENERS (WITH EXERCISE CIRCLE) ▬

roll over

This exercise targets your abs.

STARTING POSITION

Lie flat on your back with your spine imprinted.
Hold the circle between your ankles and bend
your legs at a 90-degree angle. Rest your arms at
your sides, palms down.

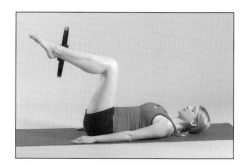

1. Reach your legs straight to a 75-degree angle.
   Inhale as you contract your abs, keeping your
   legs extended. Use your abs to lift your tailbone and start to bring your legs overhead.

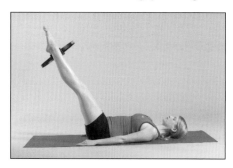
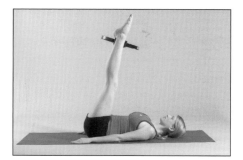

2. Exhale and squeeze the circle as you roll
   back on your shoulders and bring your
   legs all the way over your head until your
   toes are touching the floor. Avoid rolling
   onto your neck.

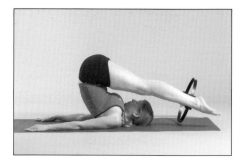

3. Inhale and release the tension on the circle as you lift your legs until they are parallel with the floor.

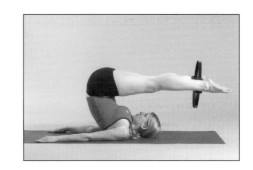

4. Squeeze the circle as you exhale and roll your spine back down onto the mat, returning your legs to the 90-degree Starting Position. Release the tension on the circle.

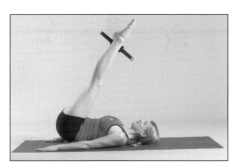
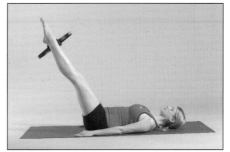

Repeat 10 times.

tip

from your personal trainer

➤ If you have a bad neck, skip this exercise or perform the modified version below.
➤ Remember to keep your arms and palms resting on the floor.
➤ Do not throw your legs over your head. A slow, steady motion is the key to rolling along the center of your spine.

TO MODIFY:
Do not roll back on your shoulders. Roll your tailbone just off the mat and focus on using your lower abs.

TO INTENSIFY:
At Starting Position, lower your legs closer to the mat.

47

CORE STRENGTHENERS (WITH EXERCISE CIRCLE) ▬

rolling like a ball

This exercise massages your back and builds abdominal strength.

STARTING POSITION

Sit with your legs together, knees bent, and hands holding the circle just in front of your shins. Form yourself into a ball by curving your spine. Shift your weight back off your sit bones, lift your feet just off the mat, and balance.

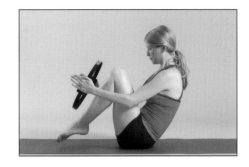

1. Inhale and roll back onto the mat, maintaining the C-curve of your spine and the contraction of your abs.

2. Exhale and squeeze the circle as you roll back up without changing the ball shape of your body. Release the tension on the circle.

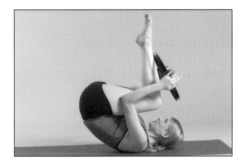

Repeat 10 times.

tip from your personal trainer

➤ Roll down the center of your spine.
➤ Be sure not to roll back on your neck.
➤ Do not use your legs for momentum. Keep yourself rolled up in a ball and let your abs do the work.

TO MODIFY:

Skip the roll and hold your balance in Starting Position for 5 breaths.

saw

Use this exercise to stretch your hamstrings and lower back.

STARTING POSITION

Begin sitting tall, with your legs stretched out in front of you at shoulder width and your feet flexed. With the circle between your hands, extend your arms out in front of you.

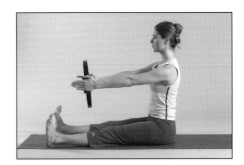

1. Inhale and twist at your waist until your inner arm is just past your leg.

2. Squeeze the circle as you exhale and roll from your head down, reaching toward your little toe.

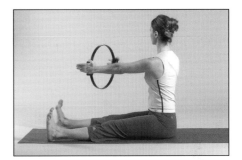

3. Inhale and release the tension on the circle as you tighten your abs and roll up through the spine.

4. Exhale and rotate back to center.

Repeat 3 times in each direction.

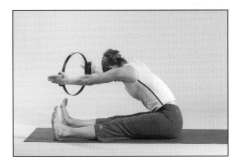

tip

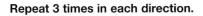
from your personal trainer

Do not move your hips or legs. Your buttocks should stay glued to the mat.

TO MODIFY:
Sit on a pillow to help stay up on your sit bones.

CORE STRENGTHENERS (WITH EXERCISE CIRCLE) ■

one-leg stretch

This exercise increases your coordination, tightens your buttocks and abs, and lengthens the muscles in your legs and hips.

STARTING POSITION

Lie flat on your back with your spine imprinted. Lift your legs and bend your knees at a 90-degree angle. Hold the circle between your hands and stretch your arms straight up.

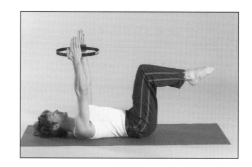

1. Inhale and center yourself.

2. Exhale and lift your upper body off the mat.

3. Inhale again, holding your position.

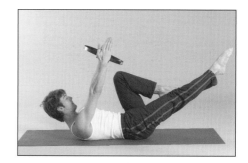

4. Exhale and squeeze the circle, extending your right leg horizontal to the mat.

5. Release the tension on the circle as you inhale and start to bring your right leg back to Starting Position while extending your left leg horizontal to the mat.

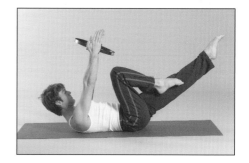

6. Exhale and squeeze the circle as you fully extend your left leg horizontal to the mat.

7. Inhale and release the tension on the circle as you begin to switch leg positions again.

Repeat 10 times.

from your personal trainer

➤ Just move your legs during this exercise. Keep your torso steady.
➤ Concentrate on extending your legs to their maximum.

TO MODIFY:
Raise your legs higher. Or keep your head on the mat and just work your legs.

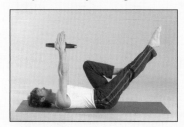

TO INTENSIFY:
Lower your legs closer to the mat.

one-leg stretch with obliques

This exercise targets the oblique muscles in your waist.

STARTING POSITION

Lie flat on your back with your spine imprinted.
Lift your legs and bend your knees at a 90-degree
angle. Hold the circle between your hands and
stretch your arms straight up.

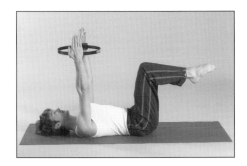

1. Center yourself with an inhale and nod
   your chin.

2. Exhale to lift your body off the mat and
   squeeze the circle while simultaneously extending your right leg out straight and rotating your
   upper body toward your bent left knee.

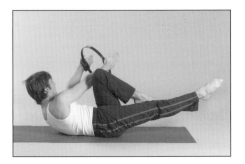

3. Inhale and release the tension on the circle
   while you rotate your upper body back to the
   center and begin to switch leg positions.

4. Exhale and squeeze the circle while simultaneously extending your left leg out straight
   and rotating your upper body toward your
   bent right knee.

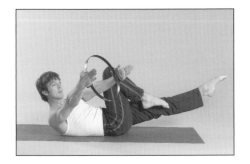

5. Release the tension on the circle and inhale
   while you rotate your upper body back to the
   center and begin to switch leg positions.

Repeat 10 times.

HOT BOD FUSION

TO MODIFY:

Keep your feet on the floor and just move your upper body. Spine is neutral.

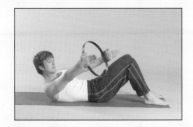

TO INTENSIFY:

Lower your legs closer to the mat while maintaining your imprint.

double leg stretch

Use this move to tone your abs and thighs.

STARTING POSITION

Lie flat on your back with your spine imprinted. Lift your legs and bend your knees at a 90-degree angle. Place the circle between your ankles and your hands behind your head.

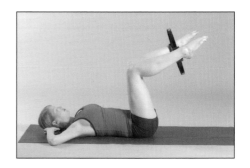

1. Inhale and center yourself.

2. Nod your chin to your chest as you exhale and flex your spine. Simultaneously reach your legs out as low as you are comfortable without touching the mat.

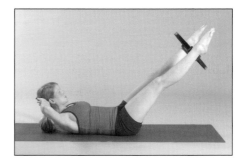

3. Inhale again and hold.

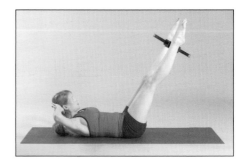

4. Then lift your legs toward the ceiling (high, higher, and highest at 90 degrees) and squeeze and release the circle in three short pulses. Exhale on each pulse.

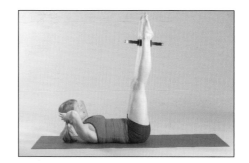

5. Keeping your chin to your chest, inhale, and bend your knees to a 90-degree angle.

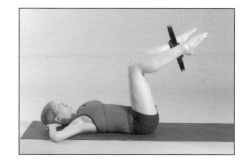

6. Exhale and lower your head back to the mat.

Repeat 6 times.

tip **from your personal trainer**

TO MODIFY:
Raise your legs higher. Or keep your head on the mat.

TO INTENSIFY:
Lower your legs closer to the mat.

CORE STRENGTHENERS (WITH EXERCISE CIRCLE) ■

mid-back extension

This exercise improves your posture and strengthens your back muscles.

STARTING POSITION

Lie flat on your stomach, with your knees bent at 90 degrees. Place the circle between your ankles, and then place your hands at your waist with your palms down.

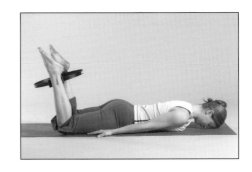

1. Inhale and squeeze the circle as you lift your chest and head off the mat.

2. Exhale and release the tension on the circle as you lower your chest and head back down to mat.

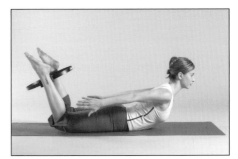

Repeat 6 times.

tip **from your personal trainer**

Keep your abs tight to support your lower back.

TO MODIFY:
Stay on your stomach and just squeeze the circle.

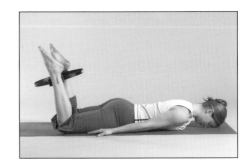

HOT BOD FUSION

spinal release

Use this counter-stretch to release and relax your spine. You don't need to use the circle for this move.

STARTING POSITION

Begin lying flat on your stomach with your arms stretched out in front of you.

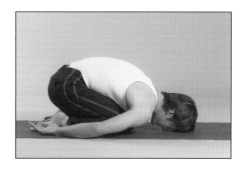

1. Push back with your hands and arms until your hips are resting on your heels. Keep your forehead on the mat and round your spine. Let your arms relax by your sides and breathe normally for several breaths.

teaser

This classic Pilates exercise is one of the most challenging workouts for your abdominal muscles.

STARTING POSITION

Begin lying on your back with your spine neutral. Put your feet on the floor, legs together, knees bent. With the circle between your hands, stretch your arms out behind your head.

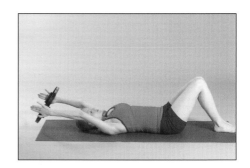

1. Slowly raise your arms as you inhale. When your fingers are pointing at the ceiling, drop your chin to your chest.

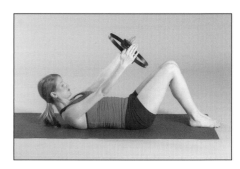

2. Exhale and squeeze the circle as you continue your forward arm motion. Peel your spine off the mat one vertebra at a time until you are sitting upright on your sit bones and your arms are just above your knees.

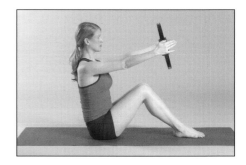

58

3. Release the tension on the circle as you inhale and raise your arms until they are just above your line of sight.

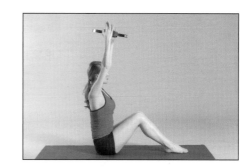

4. Exhale and squeeze the circle as you roll back down onto the mat one vertebra at a time, through the imprint, finishing with your spine neutral and your arms behind your head in Starting Position.

Repeat 6 times.

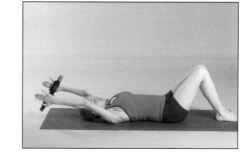

tip **from your personal trainer**

TO INTENSIFY:
Begin and finish with an imprinted spine. Place the circle between your ankles and lift your legs up to a 75-degree angle for the full exercise.

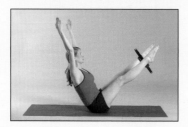

CORE STRENGTHENERS (WITH EXERCISE CIRCLE) ■

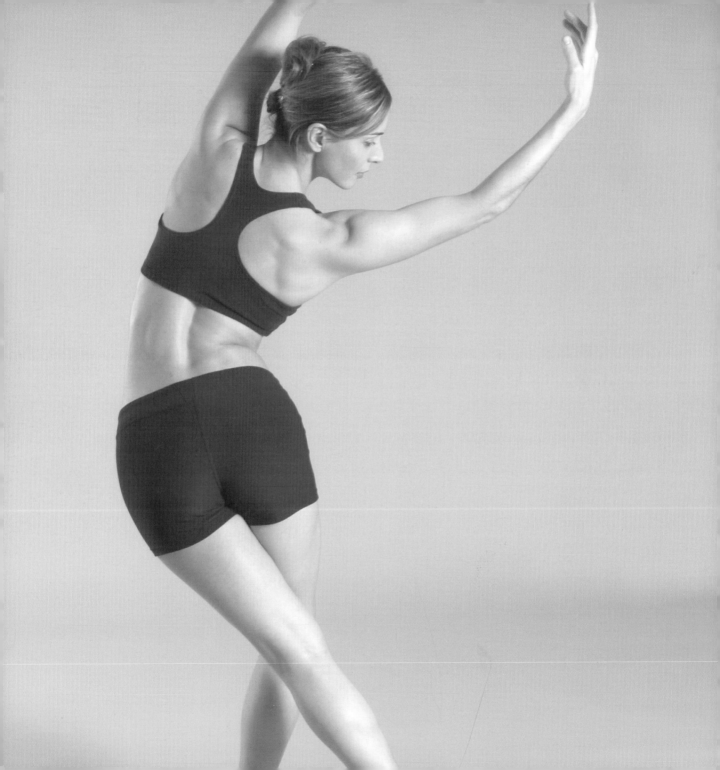

five

BOOTY TONERS

BALLET

HIS TEN-MINUTE workout uses the grace and poise of ballet as an overall stretch for the entire body, and specifically to tone your tush, thighs, and abs. Remember not to rush your movements. Concentrate on your form.

ARM MOVEMENTS

If you are ready to add an even more challenging element to your ballet workout, follow the arm movements in the photographs. If not, just leave them out.

BREATHING

Relax and breathe normally during the ballet exercises. Concentrate on incorporating your breathing as a natural extension of your movements. In general, inhale as you prepare for a movement and exhale as you perform the movement.

plié into relevé (feet in first position)

This exercise will tone your tush and inner thighs.

STARTING POSITION

Begin with your feet in First Position (see page 8 to refresh your memory on correct foot placement). Stand sideways to the back of a chair or table that comes to about hip level (or a ballet barre, if you have access to one!). Place one hand lightly on the chair for support. Hold your other arm low.

First begin with a simple plié:

1. Bend your knees sideways and out over your toes.

2. Return to Starting Position.

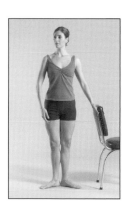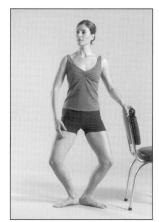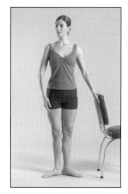

Repeat 8 times.

Then move on to the plié into relevé:

plié into relevé **(feet in first position)** *(continued)*

1. Bend your knees sideways and out over your toes.

2. Return to Starting Position.

3. Lift your heels and press onto your toes.

4. Return to Starting Position.

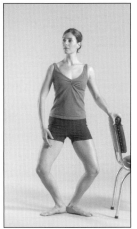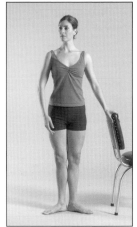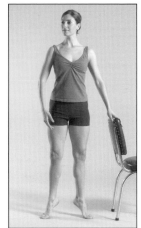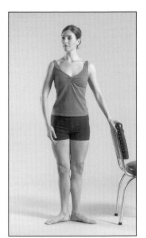

Repeat 8 times. Switch sides and repeat entire sequence.

from your personal trainer

- ➤ Don't turn your toes out too far. You should be able to align your knees over your toes during the plié.
- ➤ Point your knees out over your toes as opposed to pointing them forward.
- ➤ Your stomach should be pulled in, and your backside should not stick out.
- ➤ Stay tall and lifted throughout the entire movement.
- ➤ Continue down in the plié as far as you can without lifting you heels.
- ➤ For the relevé, keep your legs straight and turned out. Squeeze your buttocks.

TO MODIFY:

Leave out the arm movement.
Keep your hand on your hip.

TO INTENSIFY:

Finish your last relevé by balancing without holding on to the back of the chair.

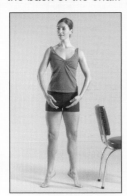

plié into relevé (feet in second position)

This exercise will tone your tush and inner thighs.

STARTING POSITION

Arrange your feet in Second Position (see page 8 to refresh your memory on correct foot placement). Stand sideways to the back of a chair that comes to about hip level. Place one hand lightly on the chair for support. Hold your other arm low.

Begin with a simple plié:

1. Bend your knees sideways and out over your toes.

2. Return to Starting Position.

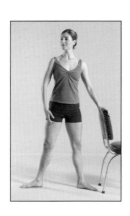 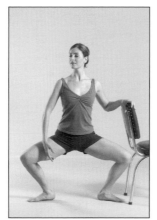 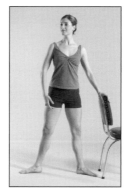

Repeat 8 times.

Then move on to the plié into relevé:

1. Bend your knees sideways and out over your toes.

2. Return to Starting Position.

3. Lift your heels and press onto your toes.

4. Return to Starting Position.

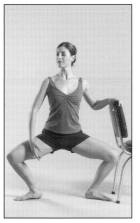 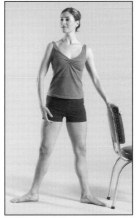 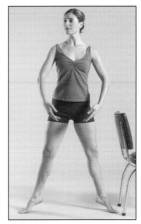 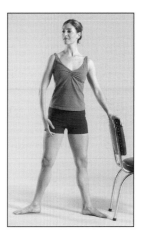

Repeat 8 times. Switch sides and repeat entire sequence.

tip **from your personal trainer**

TO INTENSIFY:
On your last relevé, balance without holding onto the back of the chair.

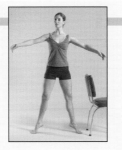

cambres

This is a wonderfully fluid, overall stretch for your body.

STARTING POSITION

Begin with your feet in First Position. Stand sideways to a chair with a back that reaches about hip level. Place one hand lightly on the back of the chair for support. Raise your other arm and round it over your head.

1. Lifting up and out of your hips, bend forward until your back is parallel to the floor.

2. Reach your nose to your knees by rounding your spine forward.

3. Straighten your spine and come back up to Starting Position.

4. Look over your shoulder toward your raised arm as you extend your spine back.

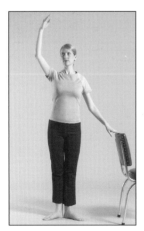 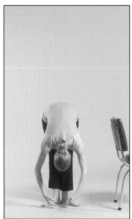 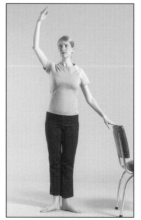 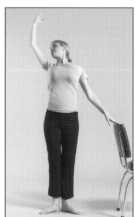

5. Return to Starting Position.

6. Reach your raised arm toward the chair as you bend sideways for a lateral stretch.

7. Straighten back up to center and perform a lateral stretch in the opposite direction, reversing the position of your arm as you do so.

8. Return to Starting Position.

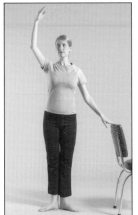 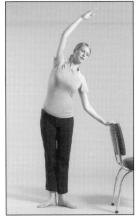 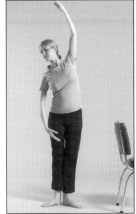 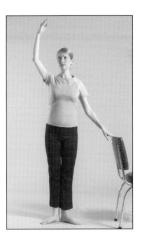

Repeat 3 times and change sides. Repeat entire sequence 4 times on each side.

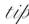 *tip* **from your personal trainer**

➤ When you first bend forward from the hips, you should keep your back long and straight, parallel to the floor.
➤ Remember to let your head relax and drop forward when you bend forward.
➤ During the back extension, be careful not to lose control of your center. Only bend back as far as you are comfortable, with your abs pulled in.

tendu/tendu and flex

This exercise will strengthen and warm your foot.

STARTING POSITION

Arrange your feet in First Position. Stand sideways to a chair and place one hand lightly on the chair back for support. Hold your other arm low or round it over your head.

First begin with tendu:

1. Slide your outside foot forward and point your foot until your big toe is just touching the floor. Return your foot to Starting Position and repeat 4 times.

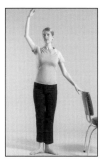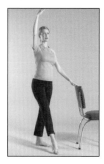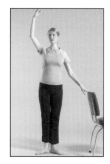

2. Sweep your leg out to the side and point your foot until your big toe is just touching the floor, heel facing the front to keep your leg turned out. Return your foot to Starting Position and repeat 4 times.

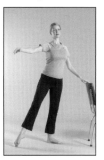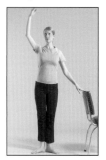

HOT BOD FUSION

3. Sweep your foot backward and point your foot until your big toe is just touching the floor. Return your foot to Starting Position and repeat 4 times.

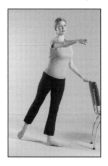 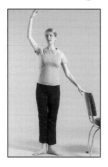

4. Sweep your leg out to the side and point your foot until your big toe is just touching the floor, heel facing the front to keep your leg turned out. Return your foot to Starting Position and repeat 4 times.

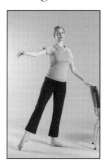 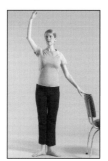

5. Plié to finish.

Then move on to the tendu and flex:

tendu/tendu and flex *(continued)*

1. Slide your outside foot forward and point your foot until your big toe is just touching the floor. Flex your foot and then return your big toe to the floor. Return your foot to Starting Position and repeat 4 times.

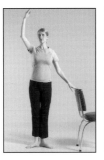 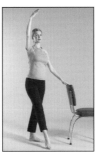 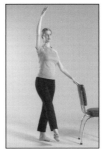 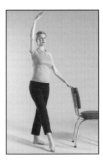 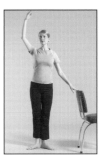

2. Sweep your leg out to the side and point your foot until your big toe is just touching the floor. Flex your foot and then return your big toe to the floor. Return your foot to Starting Position and repeat 4 times.

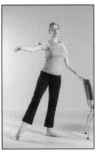 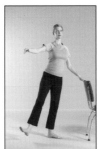 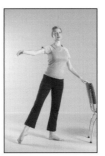 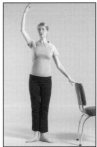

3. Sweep your foot backward and point your foot until your big toe is just touching the floor. Flex your foot and then return your big toe to the floor. Return your foot to Starting Position and repeat 4 times.

HOT BOD FUSION

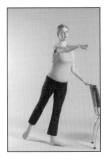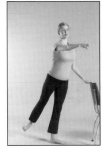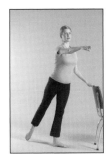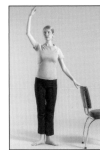

4. Sweep your leg out to the side and point your foot until your big toe is just touching the floor. Flex your foot and then return your big toe to the floor. Return your foot to Starting Position and repeat 4 times.

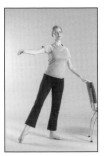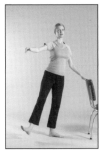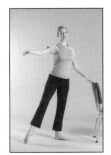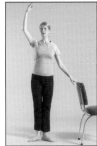

5. Plié to finish.

Switch sides and repeat entire sequence.

tip **from your personal trainer**

➤ Your toes should never leave the floor until you flex.
➤ Keep your hips squared to the front throughout this exercise.
➤ On tendu to the front (Step 1), lead with your heel to keep your leg turned out.
➤ On tendu to the back (Step 3), lead with your toe and concentrate on lining up your foot with your tailbone.

BOOTY TONERS ▬

rond de jambe

This circular movement will tone your tush and improve hip socket mobility. It is similar to tendu, but your foot moves in smooth half-circles.

STARTING POSITION

Begin with your feet in First Position. Stand sideways to a chair and place one hand lightly on the chair back for support. Raise your other arm and round it over your head.

1. Lead with your heel and stretch your leg forward in tendu, pointing your toes at the end.

2. Circle your leg to the side and then to the back, keeping your big toe pointed and touching the floor. As your foot sweeps to the back, reach your arm in front of you until it is parallel to the floor.

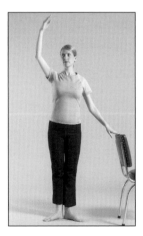 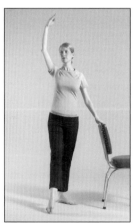 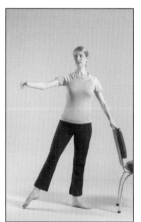 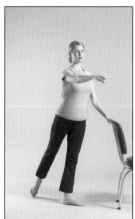

HOT BOD FUSION

3. Pull your leg back through to First Position, raising your arm back to the ceiling as you do so.

4. Return to Starting Position and continue into another rond de jambe. Repeat 4 times.

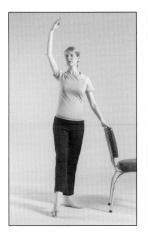 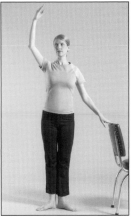

5. Reverse the direction of your leg and arm. Start by sweeping your leg to the back and finish in the front. Repeat 4 times and plié to finish.

Switch sides and repeat entire sequence.

 tip

from your personal trainer

➤ Your foot should never leave the floor.
➤ Keep your heel facing forward to maintain the outward rotation of the leg. Think of leading with the inside of your heel.
➤ Keep your hips squared to the front throughout this exercise.

TO INTENSIFY:
Increase your speed while maintaining good form.

frappé

This exercise strengthens your leg muscles.

STARTING POSITION

Arrange your feet in First Position. Stand sideways to a chair and place one hand lightly on the chair back for support. Place your other arm on your hip or round it over your head.

1. Tendu to Second Position by pointing your working leg out to the side, with your big toe just touching the floor.

2. Flex your working foot.

3. Bring the heel from your working leg to just above and in front of the ankle of the standing leg.

4. Strike your working foot out in front of you and point your foot until your big toe touches the ground.

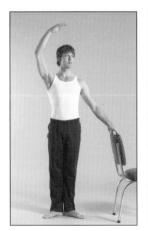 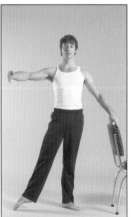 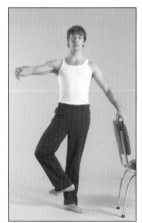 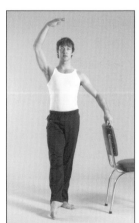

5. Return your heel to just above and in front of your ankle.

6. Repeat last two steps 8 times.

7. Now repeat 8 times to the back, this time placing your heel behind the ankle of your standing leg, toes pointing back to ensure turn-out of your leg (as pictured in the final three photographs).

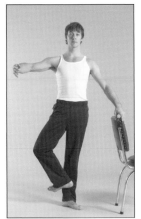 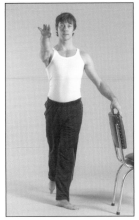 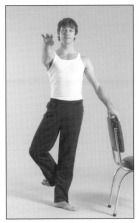 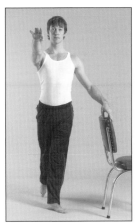

Switch sides and repeat entire sequence.

tip

from your personal trainer

➤ This is a sharp movement. Your foot should strike the floor, not sweep it.
➤ Be mindful to keep your knees pointing out, not forward.

TO INTENSIFY:
Perform the entire combination in relevé (see pages 62–63 for instructions on how to execute a relevé) and strike the air instead of the floor with your foot. You start in relevé and stay in relevé for the full 8 repetitions.

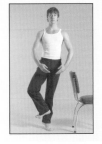

dégagé

This exercise will give your inner thighs a great workout.

STARTING POSITION

Arrange your feet in First Position. Stand sideways to a chair and place one hand lightly on the chair back for support. Raise your other arm and round it over your head.

1. Keep your center tight and your arm lifted.

2. Leading with your heel, kick your working leg out in front of you a few inches off the floor.

3. Return to Starting Position and repeat 8 times.

4. Keep your center tight, and lower your arm in front of you.

5. Leading with your heel, kick your working leg behind you a few inches off the floor.

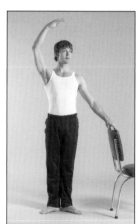

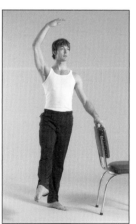
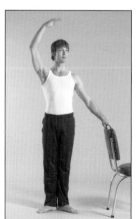
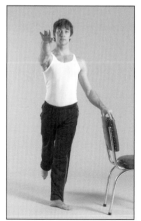

6. Repeat 8 times and plié to finish.

Switch sides and repeat entire sequence

from your personal trainer

➤ Keep your hips squared to the front throughout this exercise.
➤ As you dégagé front, concentrate on using your inner thigh, not your quadriceps.
➤ These are big energetic kicks. Kick up quickly; come down slow and controlled.
➤ Pull in from your center and stay lifted with the rest of your body.

TO INTENSIFY:
Perform the exercise without holding the chair back, using your abdominals for control.

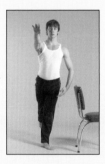

TO MODIFY:
Place your working arm on your hip.

front attitude

This exercise strengthens your leg muscles.

STARTING POSITION

Begin with your feet in First Position. Stand sideways to a chair and place one hand lightly on the chair back for support. Place your other arm low.

1. Tendu to Second Position by pointing your working leg out to the side, big toe just touching the floor.

2. Keep your toes pointed and bring your foot just above and in front of the ankle of your standing leg, knee pointing to the side. Now plié. (This is called fondu.)

3. Straighten your standing leg.

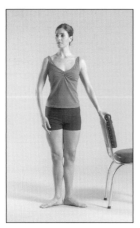 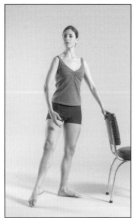 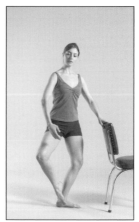 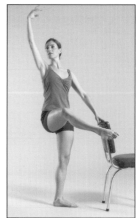

4. Lift your bent working leg out in front of you until it is parallel to the floor.

5. Return your pointed foot to just above and in front of the ankle of your standing leg.

6. Repeat the last two steps 8 times, maintaining a straight standing leg throughout.

7. Finish in First Position.

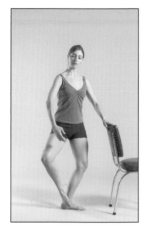 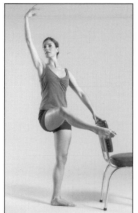 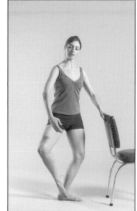 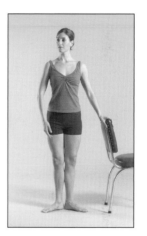

Switch sides and repeat entire sequence.

tip **from your personal trainer**

➤ Keep your hips squared to the front throughout this exercise.
➤ Be careful not to let your foot drop in the attitude.

TO INTENSIFY:
Stand away from the chair. Balance and hold the last attitude.

arabasque

This movement increases your coordination while toning your tush, hamstrings, and lower back.

STARTING POSITION

Arrange your feet in First Position. Stand sideways to a chair and place one hand lightly on the chair back for support. Place your other arm low.

1. Tendu to Second Position by pointing your working leg out to the side, big toe just touching the floor.

2. Trace a quarter circle on the floor with your big toe until your foot is directly behind you.

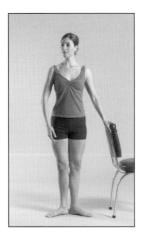
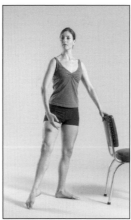
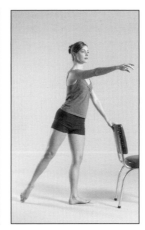

3. Lean slightly forward as you lift your working leg backward as high as possible while maintaining good form.

4. Lower your leg until your big toe just touches the ground.

5. Repeat the last two steps 8 times and finish in First Position.

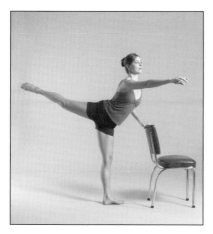 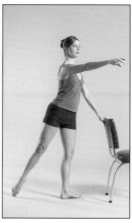 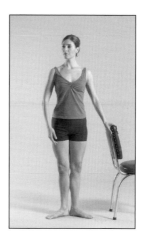

Switch sides and repeat entire sequence.

tip **from your personal trainer**

➤ Allow your upper body to move slightly forward without losing your abdominal connection.
➤ Keep your shoulders square and sliding away from your ears.

TO INTENSIFY:
Stand away from the chair. On the last arabesque, lift your leg even higher, allowing your upper body to lean forward, and begin reaching your arm for the floor. Take this as far as you can, using the height of your leg as a guide to how far you allow yourself to lean forward.

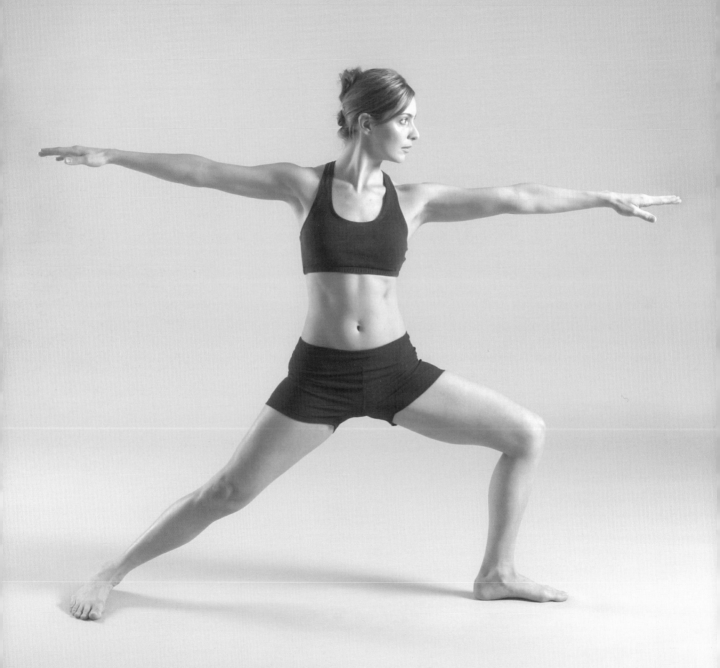

SIX

FLOWING ENERGIZERS
YOGA

HIS TEN-MINUTE workout uses the balance, agility, and strength of yoga to release tension while lengthening and strengthening your muscles. The following series of poses should flow one into the other. Aim to hold each pose for one inhale or exhale, allowing the breath and poses to flow one into the other. If this seems too speedy when you are beginning, hold each pose for more than one breath. Just keep breathing!

sun salutation (beginner)

This classic yoga series promotes flexibility in your spine and limbs.

STARTING POSITION

Stand straight, with your legs parallel and feet together. Place your arms at your sides and relax your hands.

1. **MOUNTAIN POSE:** Inhale and pull your abs toward your spine. Open your chest and relax your shoulders.

2. **FORWARD BEND:** Exhale as you roll down one vertebrae at a time and reach your hands for your feet. Ideally, you want to place your palms flat on the floor next to your feet. Tuck your head in toward your knees.

from your personal trainer

TO MODIFY FORWARD BEND: Bend your knees. Or don't reach your hands all the way to the floor.

3. **REACH FLOOR:** As your fingertips reach for the mat, inhale and lift your head and tailbone to straighten your spine, forming a line from the crown of your head to your tailbone.

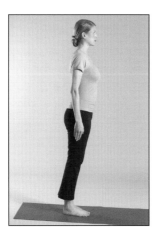
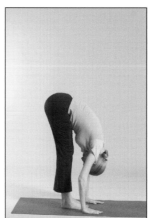
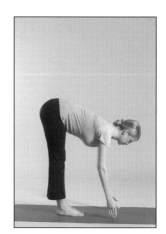

HOT BOD FUSION

4. **PLANK POSE:** Exhale, place your palms on the mat, and step one leg straight behind you. Step your other leg back and lower your hips so that your body forms a straight line from head to heels.

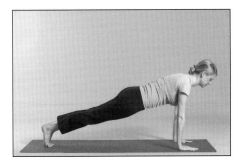

 tip **from your personal trainer**

During Plank Pose, keep your abs tight so you do not sag in the center.

TO INTENSIFY PLANK POSE:
Jump both legs back simultaneously instead of stepping back one leg at a time.

5. **UPWARD DOG:** Keeping your arms straight, inhale and let your hips come forward to the mat. Raise your face to the ceiling, extend your spine, and place the back of your feet on the mat. Slide your shoulders away from your ears.

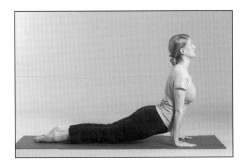

 tip **from your personal trainer**

During Upward Dog, be careful not to overextend your head and neck.

6. **DOWNWARD DOG:** Keeping your hands flat on the floor, exhale and roll back onto the bottom of your feet as you lift your hips into the air to form an inverted V.

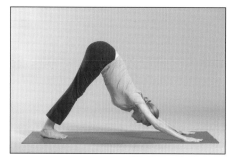

 tip **from your personal trainer**

During Downward Dog, keep your shoulders sliding away from your ears and your abs tight.

TO MODIFY DOWNWARD DOG:
Keep your knees soft and bent.

7. **FORWARD BEND:** Keeping your hands flat on the floor, inhale and step one leg forward so that your foot is between your hands. Likewise, step your other leg forward.

8. **MOUNTAIN POSE:** Exhale as you roll your spine up slowly. Inhale and pull your abs toward your spine. Exhale and center yourself.

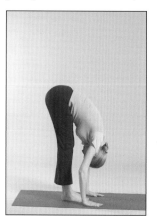 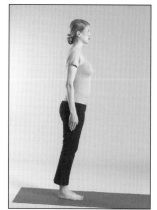

Repeat 4 times, alternating your lead leg each time.

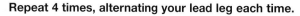

sun salutation (advanced)

This is a more intense series of poses than the Sun Salutation on page 86. Add this to your routine when you are comfortable with that Sun Salutation. You may vary the series by holding the poses longer.

STARTING POSITION

Stand straight, legs parallel and feet together. Place your arms at your sides and relax your hands.

1. **MOUNTAIN POSE:** Inhale and pull your abs toward your spine.

2. **CHAIR POSE:** Exhale as you bend both knees as if sitting in a chair. Reach your arms overhead, palms facing in.

 tip **from your personal trainer**

During Chair Pose, relax your shoulders away from your ears.

3. **REACH SKY:** Inhale and stand tall as in Mountain Pose. Reach your arms straight up as you extend your spine slightly and tighten your abs. Lift your eyes to the sky.

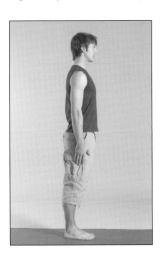 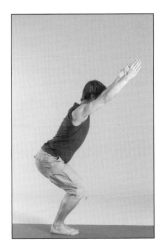 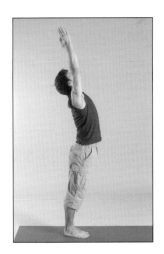

4. **FORWARD BEND:** Exhale as you roll down one vertebra at a time and reach your hands for your feet. Ideally, you want to place your palms flat on the floor next to your feet. Tuck your head in toward your knees.

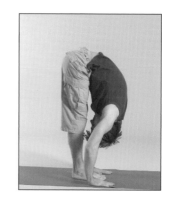

tip **from your personal trainer**

TO MODIFY FORWARD BEND:
Bend your knees, or don't reach your hands all the way to the floor

TO INTENSIFY:
Jump both legs back simultaneously instead of stepping back.

5. **REACH FLOOR:** As your fingertips reach for the mat, inhale and lift your head and tailbone to straighten your spine, forming a line from the crown of your head to your tailbone.

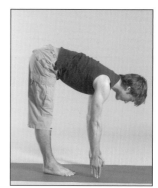

6. **PUSH-UP:** Exhale, place your palms on the mat, and step one leg straight behind you. Step your other leg back and lower your hips so that your body forms a straight line from head to heels. Tighten your abs and lower your entire body to the floor. Keep your shoulders open and your elbows close to your body.

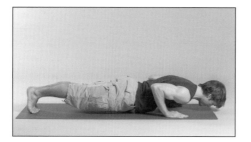

tip **from your personal trainer**

During Push-Up, be careful not to lift your tush or let your center and hips sag.

TO MODIFY PUSH-UP:
Lower your knees to the floor.

7. **UPWARD DOG:** Inhale as you straighten your arms, extend your spine, and raise your face to the ceiling. Simultaneously place the back of your pointing feet on the mat. Slide your shoulders away from your ears.

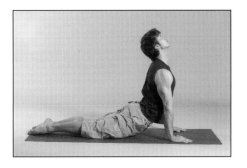

 tip **from your personal trainer**

During Upward Dog, be careful not to overextend your head and neck.

8. **DOWNWARD DOG:** Keeping your hands flat on the floor, exhale and roll back onto the bottom of your feet as you lift your hips into the air to form an inverted V.

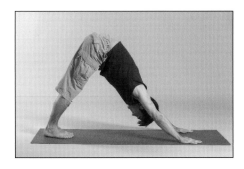

 tip **from your personal trainer**

During Downward Dog, keep your shoulders sliding away from your ears and your abs tight.

TO MODIFY DOWNWARD DOG:
Keep your knees soft and bent.

sun salutation (advanced) *(continued)*

9. **WARRIOR LUNGE RIGHT:** Inhale and step your right leg forward so that your foot is just inside your right hand. Keep your right knee bent at a 90-degree angle and aligned with your right ankle. Lift your upper body as you spread your arms out to the side and then overhead until your palms come together. Look toward your hands as you extend your spine.

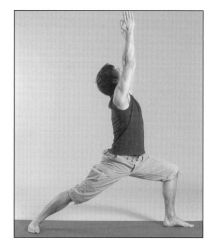

tip **from your personal trainer**

During Warrior Lunge, slide your shoulder blades down your spine.

TO MODIFY WARRIOR LUNGE:
Keep your hands on your hips and look straight ahead.

10. **PUSH-UP:** Exhale, place your palms on the mat, and step one leg straight behind you. Step your other leg back and lower your hips so that your body forms a straight line from head to heels. Tighten your abs and lower your entire body to the floor. Keep your shoulders open and your elbows close to your body.

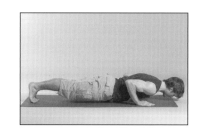

11. **UPWARD DOG:** Inhale as you straighten your arms, extend your spine, and raise your face to the ceiling. Simultaneously place the back of your pointing feet on the mat. Slide your shoulders away from your ears.

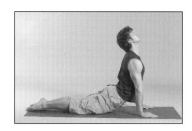

HOT BOD FUSION

12. **DOWNWARD DOG:** Keeping your hands flat on the floor, exhale and roll back onto the bottom of your feet as you lift your hips into the air to form an inverted V.

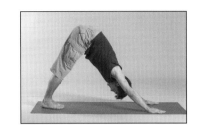

13. **WARRIOR LUNGE LEFT**: Inhale and step your left leg forward so that your foot is just inside your left hand. Keep your left knee bent at a 90-degree angle and aligned with your left ankle. Lift your upper body as you spread your arms out to the side and then overhead until your palms come together. Look toward your hands as you extend your spine.

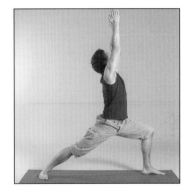

14. **PUSH-UP:** Exhale, place your palms on the mat, and step one leg straight behind you. Step your other leg back and lower your hips so that your body forms a straight line from head to heels. Tighten your abs and lower your entire body to the floor. Keep your shoulders open and your elbows close to your body.

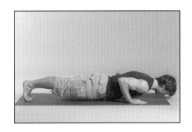

15. **UPWARD DOG:** Inhale as you straighten your arms, extend your spine, and raise your face to the ceiling. Simultaneously place the back of your pointing feet on the mat. Slide your shoulders away from your ears.

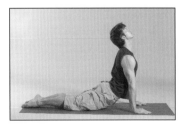

16. **DOWNWARD DOG:** Keeping your hands flat on the floor, exhale and roll back onto the bottom of your feet as you lift your hips into the air to form an inverted V.

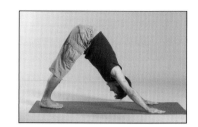

17. **REACH FLOOR:** As your fingertips reach for the mat, inhale and lift your head and tailbone to straighten your spine, forming a line from the crown of your head to your tailbone.

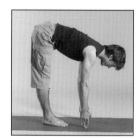

18. **FORWARD BEND:** Exhale as you roll your spine down slowly, tucking your head in toward your knees.

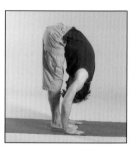

19. **REACH SKY:** Inhale and stand tall as in Mountain Pose. Reach your arms straight up as you extend your spine slightly and tighten your abs. Lift your eyes to the sky.

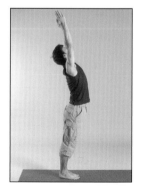

HOT BOD FUSION

20. **CHAIR POSE:** Exhale as you bend both knees as if sitting in a chair. Reach your arms overhead, palms facing in.

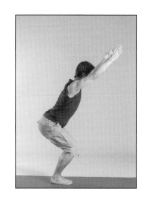

21. **MOUNTAIN POSE:** Inhale as you stand tall and pull your abs toward your spine.

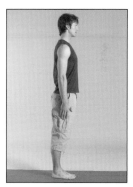

Repeat 4 times, alternating your lead leg each time.

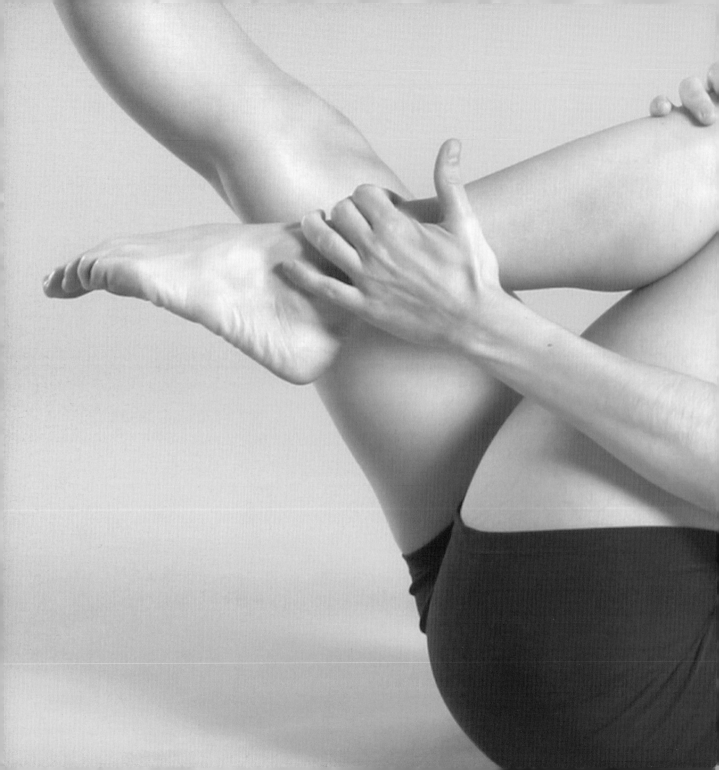

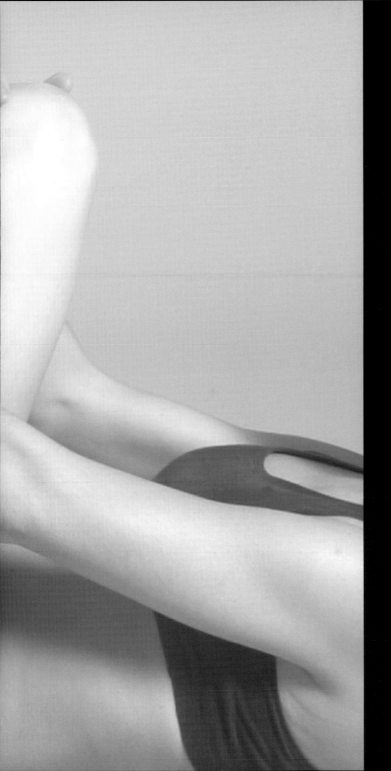

phase three

TOTAL-BODY TARGETERS

(Ten-minute workout)
Choose either Chapter 7, 8, 9, or 10

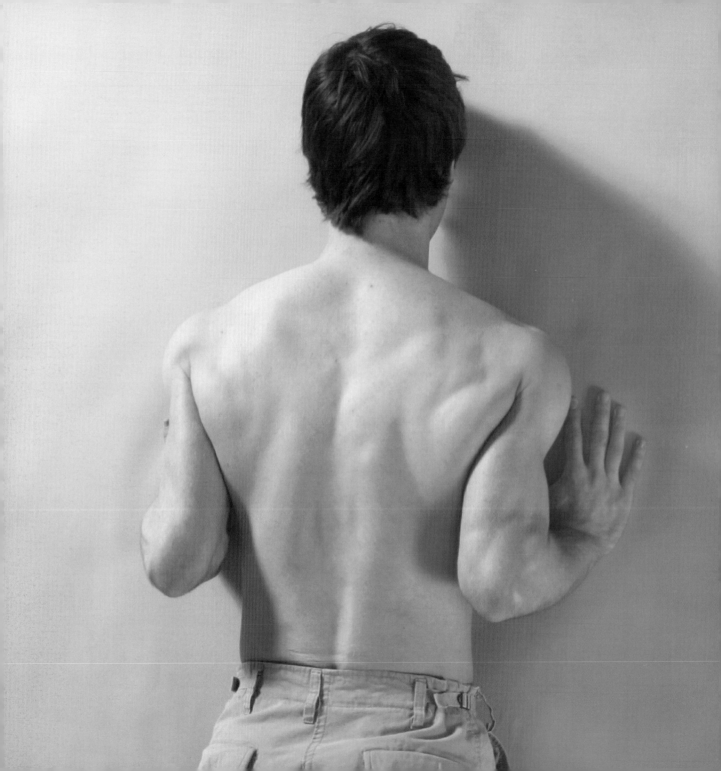

seven

TUSH TIGHTENERS
AND ARM DEFINERS

PILATES

*t*HIS TEN-MINUTE routine targets the hard-to-reach outer and inner thigh areas, the glutes, and the arms. Repeat the first five exercises on one side, then switch and repeat the sequence on the opposite side.

kick front/kick back

This exercise will stretch the back of your legs and tone up your glutes.

STARTING POSITION

Begin lying on your side with your shoulders and hips stacked on top of each other. Angle your legs about a foot in front of you, with your top leg elevated in line with your hip.

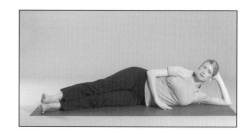

1. Inhale as you flex your top foot, sweep your leg forward as far as you can without losing your form, and pulse your leg twice.

2. Exhale and sweep your leg back behind you and point your foot.

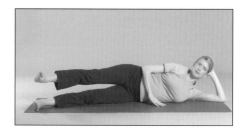

Repeat 8 times.

tip **from your personal trainer**

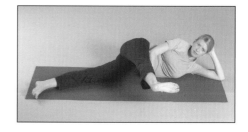

To avoid pitching your upper body forward, keep your abs contracted and your hips stacked.

TO INTENSIFY:
Place both hands behind your head. This will challenge your core stability even more.

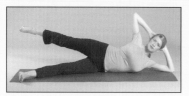

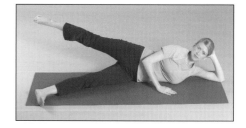

point up, flex down

This move targets the hard-to-reach outer thigh, as well as stretches the foot.

STARTING POSITION

Lie on your side with your legs stacked. Your body should be in one long line from head to toe. Rest your head on your bottom hand, and rest your top hand in front of you at chest level.

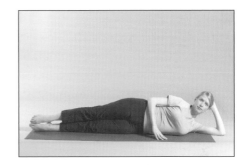

1. Inhale while you point your top foot and lift your leg to shoulder height.

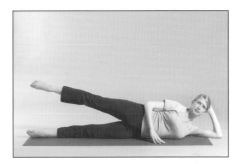

2. Flex your foot and exhale as you pull your top leg back down.

Repeat 8 times.

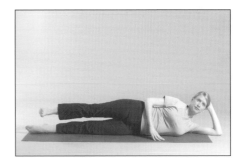

 tip **from your personal trainer**

TO INTENSIFY:
Place both hands behind your head.

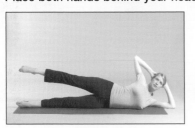

oblique flexion

This exercise will help you keep your waistline slender.

STARTING POSITION

Lie on your side with your legs stacked. Your body should be in one long line from head to toe. Rest your head on your bottom arm, which is flat on the mat for stability, and rest your top arm down the side of your body.

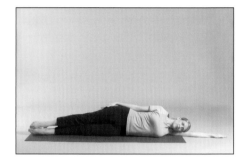

1. Inhale and simultaneously lift your upper body and legs off the mat, sliding your top hand down your side toward your toes. Squeeze your legs together, keeping your inner thighs connected.

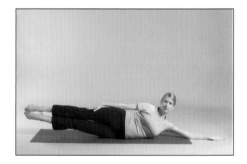

2. Exhale and return your upper body and legs to the mat.

Repeat 8 times.

tip **from your personal trainer**

Initiate the movement from your obliques. Be sure to keep your shoulders sliding down.

TO MODIFY:
Lift only your legs.

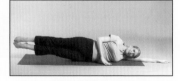

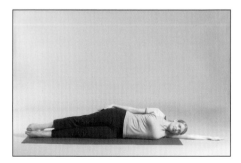

small circles

This exercise is perfect for opening the hip socket.

STARTING POSITION

Lie on your side with your legs stacked. Your body should be in one long line from head to toe. Rest your head on your bottom arm, and rest your top hand in front of you at chest level.

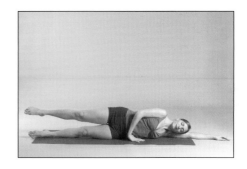

1. Lift your top leg to hip level. Breathe naturally and trace a cantaloupe-sized circle 10 times in one direction.

2. Then reverse direction and repeat 10 times.

tip **from your personal trainer**

Concentrate on just moving your leg within your hip socket and keeping the rest of your body perfectly still.

TUSH TIGHTENERS AND ARM DEFINERS ▬

large circles

This move will shape your glutes and strengthen the muscles around your hip socket.

STARTING POSITION

Lie on your side with your legs stacked. Your body should be in one long line from head to toe. Rest your head on your bottom arm, and rest your top hand in front of you at chest level.

1. Lift your top leg to hip level. Breathe naturally and trace a beach ball-sized circle 10 times in one direction.

2. Then reverse direction and repeat 10 times.

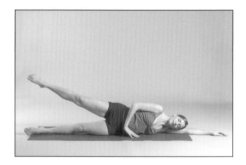

➤REMINDER: Go back and repeat the first five exercises on your other side before proceeding.

leg pull down

This exercise is both a leg and an arm toner. You will also work your abdominals to prevent torso rotation.

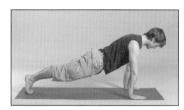

STARTING POSITION

Begin in a push-up position, abs lifting, glutes squeezing, and your body in one long line. Hips are drawn down, not lifted. Squeeze your legs together.

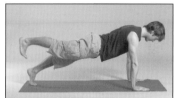

1. Raise one leg off the mat with an inhale, foot flexed.

2. Exhale and shift back onto the ball of your foot, pointing your lifted foot.

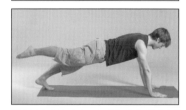

3. Lift your heel back up as you inhale and flex the foot of the lifted leg.

4. Exhale and replace the lifted leg, lower your knees to the mat, and then repeat on the other side.

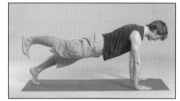

Repeat 2 to 3 times on each side.

tip

from your personal trainer

TO MODIFY:
Kneel in a push-up position. Exhale to lift the knees off the mat 2 to 4 inches and hold for 2 full breaths. Repeat 6 times.

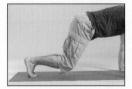

TO INTENSIFY:
Stay in Starting Position between sets—do not lower yourself to your knees.

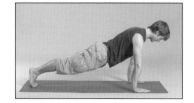

TUSH TIGHTENERS AND ARM DEFINERS ▄▄▄

roll down push-ups

Push-ups are an ideal way to tone your whole body—especially your arms and chest.

STARTING POSITION

Start standing with your legs together and arms reaching long by your sides.

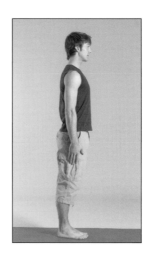 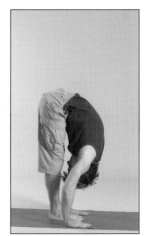

1. Inhale, drop your chin, and continue to roll down one vertebra at a time until your hands reach the mat. Bend your knees if you need to.

2. Exhale and walk your hands forward on 4 counts, stopping in a long line, ready for a push-up.

3. Inhale to lower down, exhale to push up for 5 push-ups. Inhale to walk in on 4 counts.

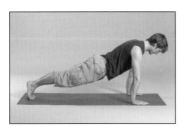 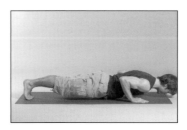 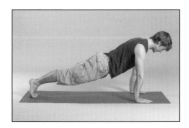

4. Exhale and slowly roll up one vertebra at a time.

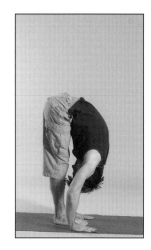 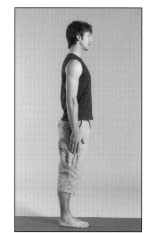

Repeat 3 times.

 tip

from your personal trainer

➤ Recall from the previous exercise that your body is in one long line before beginning the push-up.
➤ Take the roll down and roll up slowly, enjoying the stretch in your spine.

TO MODIFY:
Come to your knees for the push-ups.

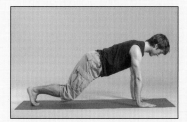

TO INTENSIFY:
Lift one leg during the push-ups.

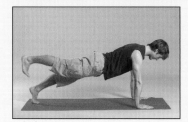

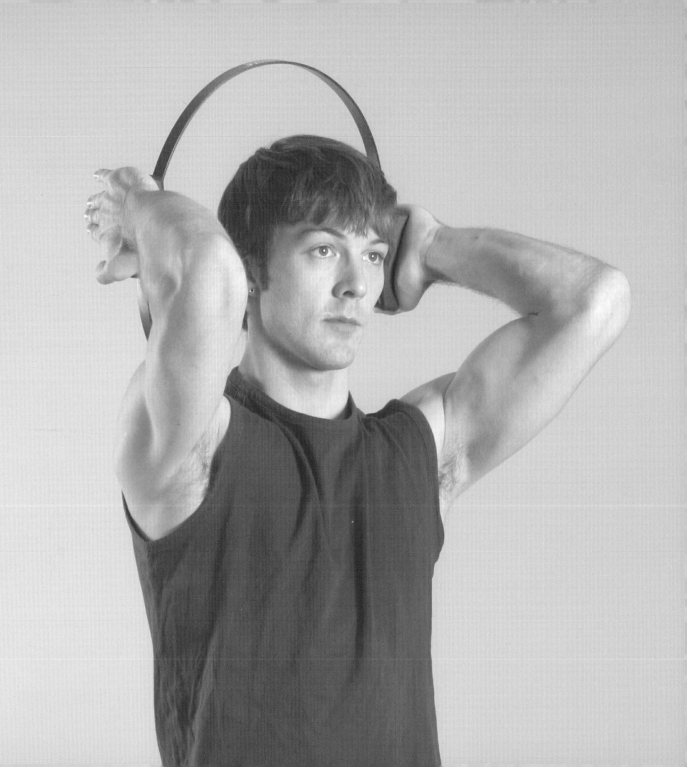

TUSH TIGHTENERS
AND ARM DEFINERS
(WITH EXERCISE CIRCLE)

PILATES

*t*HIS TEN-MINUTE workout combines classic Pilates movements with an exercise circle to tone up your tush and add definition to your arms and legs. The key is to squeeze the circle evenly (not in jerky motions), and equally (not favoring one side of your body). Do the first three exercises in this series and then switch to your other side and perform them again.

top leg inner thigh

This exercise will tone your hard-to-reach inner thighs.

STARTING POSITION

Lying on your side, place the circle between your ankles, with your bottom ankle on the inside of the circle and your top ankle on the outside of the circle. Rest your head on your bottom hand, which is stretched out horizontally with your body. Rest your top hand on the mat in front of you at chest level.

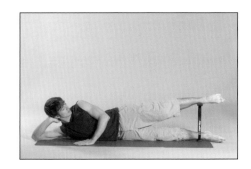

1. Inhale and center yourself.

2. Exhale and squeeze the circle slowly with your top leg.

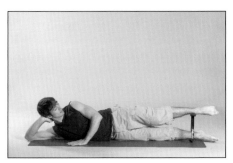

3. Inhale and release the tension on the circle.

Repeat 10 times with slow squeezes.
Repeat 10 times with quick pulses.
Repeat 5 times with slow squeezes.
Repeat 10 times with quick pulses.

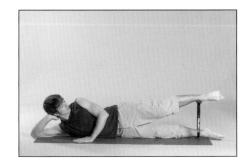

tip **from your personal trainer**

➤ Be sure not to pitch or roll your body forward or backward.
➤ Keep your legs straight, hips stacked.

HOT BOD FUSION

top leg outer thigh

This move will tighten your outer thighs and tush.

STARTING POSITION

Lying on your side, place the circle between your ankles, with your bottom ankle on the inside bottom of the circle and your top ankle on the inside top of the circle. Rest your head on your bottom hand, which is stretched out horizontally with your body. Rest your top hand on the mat in front of you at chest level.

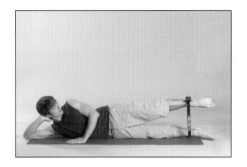

1. Inhale and center yourself.

2. Exhale and press up on the circle.

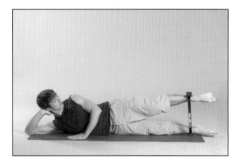

3. Inhale and release the tension on the circle.

Repeat 10 times with slow squeezes.
Repeat 10 times with quick pulses.
Repeat 5 times with slow squeezes.
Repeat 10 times with quick pulses.

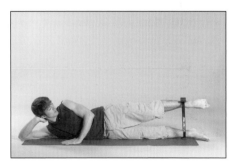

TUSH TIGHTENERS AND ARM DEFINERS (WITH EXERCISE CIRCLE) ▬

top leg rest, bottom leg lift

Doing this exercise will reward you with shapely thighs.

STARTING POSITION

Lying on your side, place the circle between your ankles, with your bottom ankle on the inside of the circle and your top ankle on the outside of the circle. Rest your head on your bottom hand, which is stretched out horizontally with your body. Rest your top hand on the mat in front of you at chest level.

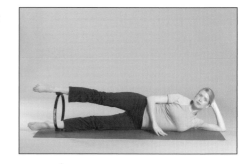

1. Inhale and center yourself.

2. Exhale and lift your bottom leg up to meet your top leg. Feel your inner thighs connect.

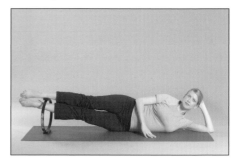

3. Lower your bottom leg back down as you inhale.

Repeat 12 times.

REMINDER: Now switch sides and repeat the first three exercises.

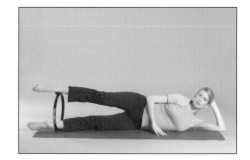

tip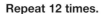
from your personal trainer

Keep your toes pointed so that your foot does not form a sickle shape.

glute squeeze

Use this to exercise to work your hamstrings and your tush.

STARTING POSITION

Lie on your stomach with your knees bent at 90 degrees. Place the circle between your ankles. Stack your hands under your forehead.

1. Inhale and center yourself.

2. Exhale and squeeze the circle.

3. Inhale and release the tension on the circle.

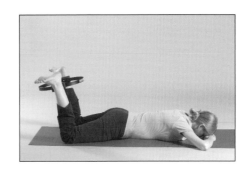

Repeat 10 times with slow squeezes.
Repeat 10 times with quick pulses.

tip **from your personal trainer**

➤ Remember to engage your abs during this movement.
➤ Squeeze the circle with equal pressure from both legs.

arms standing

This move will add definition to your arms. There are four different arm positions—make sure to do them all.

STARTING POSITION

Stand tall with your legs together.
Hold the circle between your hands.

TOP

1. Inhale and reach your arms toward the ceiling.

2. Exhale and squeeze the circle.

3. Inhale and release the tension on the circle.

Repeat 5 times.

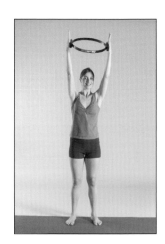

CENTER

1. Inhale and lower the circle to chest level.

2. Exhale and squeeze the circle.

3. Inhale and release the tension on the circle.

Repeat 5 times.

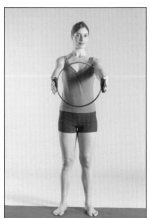

LOWER

1. Inhale and lower the circle so that it is just in front of your thighs.

2. Exhale and squeeze the circle.

3. Inhale and release the tension on the circle.

Repeat 5 times.

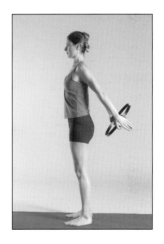

BEHIND

1. Inhale and bring the circle behind your buttocks, arms still reaching long.

2. Exhale and squeeze the circle.

3. Inhale and release the tension on the circle.

Repeat 5 times.

Repeat entire sequence 2 times.

 tip

from your personal trainer

Keep your fingers relaxed and don't bend your elbows to force the squeeze.

TUSH TIGHTENERS AND ARM DEFINERS (WITH EXERCISE CIRCLE) ■

triceps standing

This is a strength move that focuses on your triceps.

STARTING POSITION

Stand tall with your legs together. Hold the circle between your hands and lift your arms toward the ceiling.

1. Bend your elbows as you inhale and lower the circle to just behind your head.

2. Exhale and squeeze the circle as you straighten your elbows and bring the circle back in front of you.

3. Inhale and release the tension on the circle as you bend your elbows and return the circle to behind your head.

Repeat 10 times.

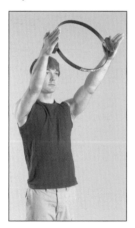 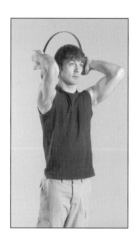 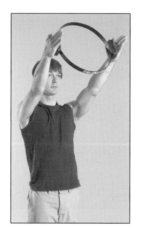 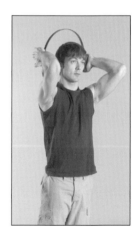

 from your personal trainer

Keep your elbows in, pointing straight out in front of your face.

plié standing

This exercise targets your tush and your inner thighs.

STARTING POSITION

Stand tall with your heels apart and your toes pointed out in a V.
Bend your knees slightly and place the circle just above your knees.

1. Inhale and center yourself.

2. Exhale as you straighten your knees slightly and squeeze the circle.

3. Return to Starting Position.

Repeat 10 times.

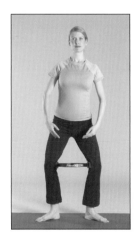 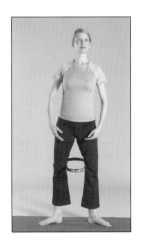 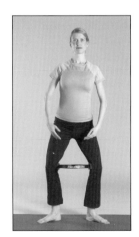 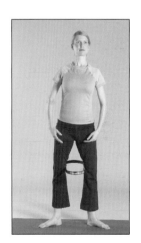

tip **from your personal trainer**

Keep your tush pulled under.

TUSH TIGHTENERS AND ARM DEFINERS (WITH EXERCISE CIRCLE)

back of leg sitting

This is another simple exercise that will tone your thighs and your tush.

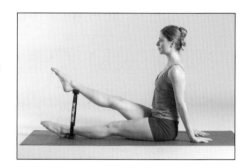

STARTING POSITION

Sit on the mat with your legs stretched straight out in front of you. Place one ankle on the inside bottom of the circle, and place the other ankle on the outside top of the circle. Sit tall and then lean back slightly as you place your hands flat on the mat behind you.

1. Inhale and center yourself.

2. Exhale and push down on the circle with your top leg.

3. Inhale and release the tension on the circle.

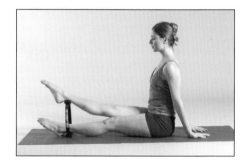

Repeat 10 times with slow squeezes.
Repeat 10 times with quick pulses.
Repeat 5 times with slow squeezes.
Repeat 10 times with quick pulses.

Repeat entire sequence with opposite leg.

tip **from your personal trainer**

Keep your top leg straight as you squeeze and release the circle. Do not bend your knee.

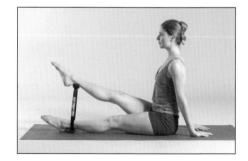

CENTER STAGE
STREAMLINERS

BALLET

*T*HIS TEN-MINUTE workout develops your balance and coordination as you take your ballet workout to a new level by stepping away from the stability of the back of a chair or a table. Don't rush your movements. Concentrate on your form.

If you are ready to add an even more challenging element to your ballet workout, follow the arm movements in the photographs. If not, just leave them out and place your hands on your hips.

dégagé combo

This fluid movement will help you achieve better balance.

STARTING POSITION

Begin with your feet in First Position. Rest your arms at your sides.

1. Shift your weight to your standing leg as you sweep your working leg out to the side and point your foot toward the ground, just lifted off the floor (dégagé).

2. Return your foot to Starting Position.

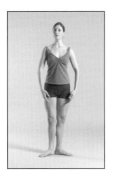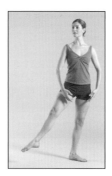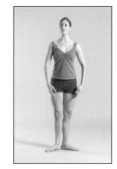

Repeat 8 times. On eighth repetition, instead of returning to Starting Position:

1. Lower your foot to the ground so that your feet are in Second Position.

2. Bend your knees (plié).

3. Remain in plié and lift your heels.

4. Staying up on your toes, straighten your legs and squeeze your glute muscles (relevé).

HOT BOD FUSION

5. Lower your heels to the ground.

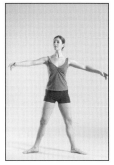 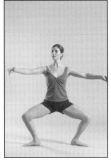 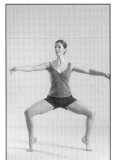 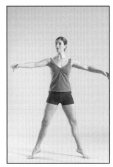 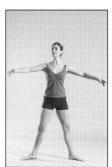

Repeat this second sequence 8 times.

TO FINISH:

1. Lift your working leg slightly and point your foot toward the ground, just lifted off the floor (dégagé).
2. Return your foot to original Starting Position.

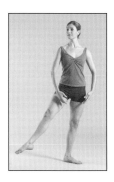 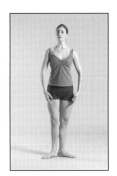

Repeat entire sequence with your opposite leg.

power plié

This exercise is a super-intense workout designed to lift your tush and slenderize your thighs.

STARTING POSITION

Arrange your feet in Second Position and stretch your arms out parallel to the floor.

1. Bend your knees (plié).

2. Remain in plié and lift your heels.

3. Staying up on your toes, straighten your legs and squeeze your glute muscles (relevé).

4. Lower your heels to return to Starting Position.

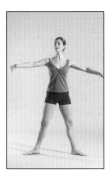 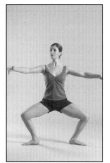 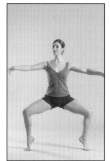 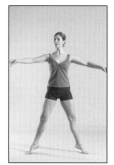 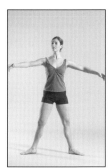

**Repeat 8 times,
then repeat 8 times in reverse
(relevé, plié,
lower your heels,
straighten your knees).**

 tip

from your personal trainer

➤ Keep your back straight and your tush pulled in during the entire exercise.
➤ Keep your knees opened outward, over your toes.

TO MODIFY:
Continue using the back of a chair or a table for balance.

HOT BOD FUSION

fondu, coupé, passé

Fondu means melting. Use this fluid movement to strengthen your legs and improve your coordination.

STARTING POSITION

Arrange your feet in First Position. Place your arms on your hips or rounded in front of you.

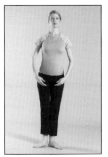 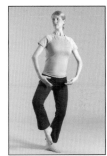

1. Sweep your working leg to the side, pointing your foot so that your toes are just touching the floor.

2. Bend (plié) your standing knee while moving your working foot to your standing ankle (coupé).

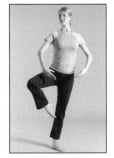 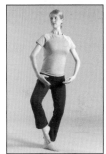

3. Straighten your standing leg while sliding your working pointed toes up your shin to your knee (passé).

4. Bend (plié) your standing knee again while sliding your working foot back down your shin to your ankle (fondu).

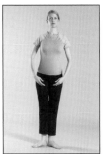

5. Return to Starting Position—legs straight, tush and inner thighs squeezing.

Repeat 10 times with each leg.

tip **from your personal trainer**

➤ Keep your working foot pointed.
➤ Keep your legs turned out throughout the entire exercise.

pirouette prep

This exercise is designed to lift your tush and slenderize your thighs.

STARTING POSITION
Arrange your feet in First Position. Place your arms on your hips or rounded in front of you.

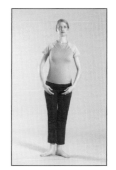

1. Sweep your working leg out to the side and point your foot until your big toe is just touching the floor, heel facing the front to keep your leg turned out (tendu second). Distribute your weight evenly between your legs.

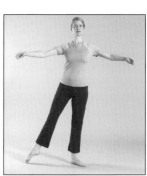

2. Keeping your weight evenly distributed, bend (plié) your knees while sweeping your working foot backward.

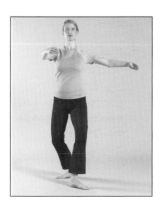

$3.$ Shift your weight to your standing leg as you straighten it. Bring your working leg forward, and slide your working pointed toe up your shin to your knee (passé).

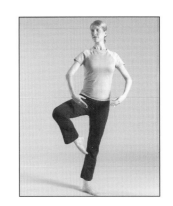

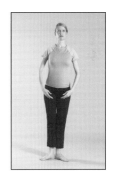

$4.$ Return to First Position.

Repeat 10 times with each leg.

tip **from your personal trainer**

In passé, keep your knee pointed out and your hips squared to the front.

TO INTENSIFY:
Balance in passé before returning to First Position. Or relevé on your standing leg as you come to passé; then balance before returning to First Position.

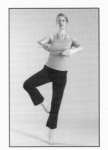

passé/dévelopé/tendu/pointe

These movements will challenge your control and stretch your legs.

STARTING POSITION

Begin with your feet in First Position. Place your arms on your hips or rounded in front of you.

1. Slide your working pointed toe up your standing shin to your knee (passé).

2. Extend your working leg straight out in front of you, leading with your heel to keep your leg turned out (dévelopé).

3. Keeping your leg straight, lower your toe to the floor (tendu).

4. Lift your leg out in front of you again (pointe).

5. Lower your foot to the floor through tendu and return to Starting Position.

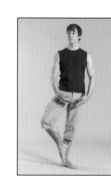
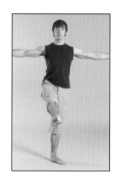
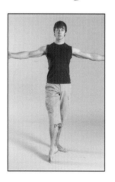
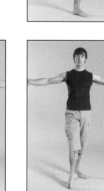
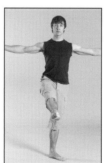
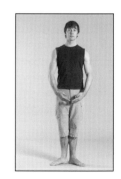

Repeat 8 times.

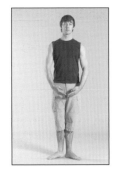 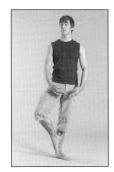

Repeat 8 more times, this time extending your
working leg straight back behind you (développé back).

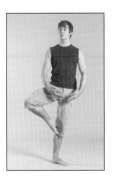 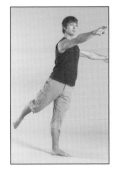 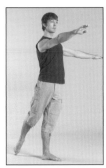 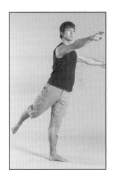

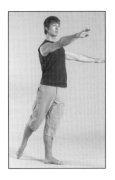 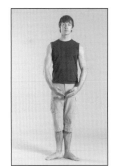

Repeat entire sequence with other leg.

 tip **from your personal trainer**

➤ This is a smooth, fluid exercise so focus on your
form, not on speed.
➤ Keep your working foot pointed.
➤ On développé back, lead with your toe in order to
maintain good turn-out of your leg.

TO MODIFY:
Keep the développé low.

TO INTENSIFY:
Lift your leg higher on développé.

CENTER STAGE STREAMLINERS ▬

back attitude

This movement will tone and strengthen the muscles surrounding your hip socket while lifting your tush and challenging your balance.

STARTING POSITION

Arrange your feet in First Position. Place your arms on your hips.

1. Sweep your working leg to the side, pointing your foot so that your toes are just touching the floor.

2. Bend (plié) your standing knee while moving your working foot so that it is just behind your right ankle (fondu).

3. Straighten your standing leg while sliding your working toe up your shin to just behind your knee (passé).

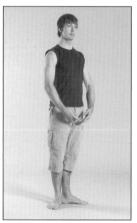 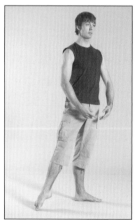 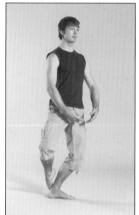 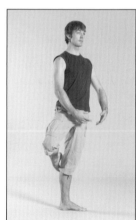

4. Keeping your working knee bent, lift your working leg up and to the back while straightening your standing leg (attitude).

5. Bend your standing knee while you lower your toe to your ankle.

6. Lift and lower your working leg 12 times to attitude, leading with the knee, toe in line with your knee.

7. Return to First Position.

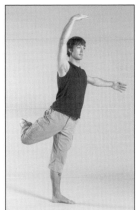 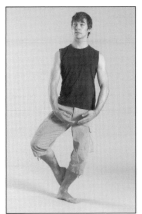 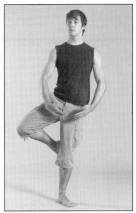 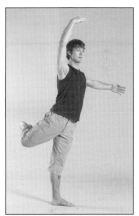

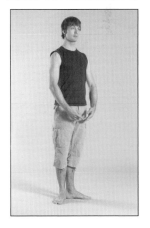

Repeat entire sequence with other leg.

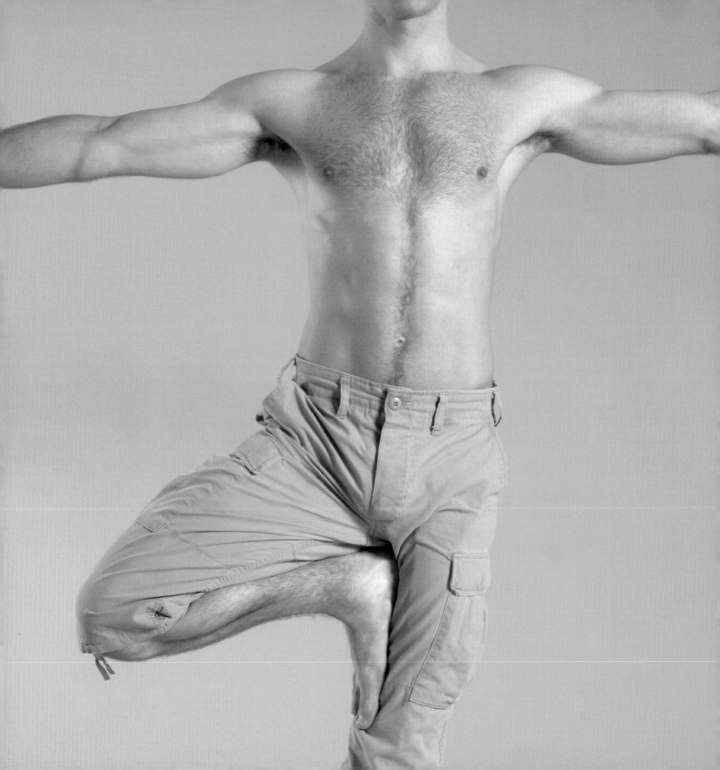

ten

BALANCE
CHALLENGERS

YOGA

THIS TEN-MINUTE workout is designed to sharpen your internal balance. It will also stretch your hamstrings and spine, build your lower body strength, and open your hips. This series of poses should flow one into the other. Aim to hold each pose for five breaths, but don't stress if you can't make it that long. Just keep breathing!

ease pose

This exercise is designed to improve your coordination and stretch your lower back.

STARTING POSITION

Begin in Mountain Pose—stand straight, legs and toes together, heels slightly apart. Place your arms at your sides and relax your hands. Inhale and pull your abs toward your spine.

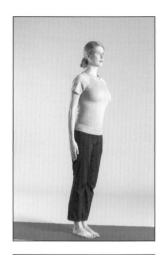

1. Bend one knee into your chest as high as possible, grasping your hands under your thigh.

2. Hold for 5 breaths.

Repeat with other leg.

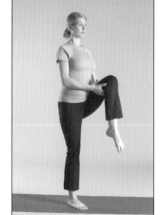

tip **from your personal trainer**

➤ Spread your toes for balance.
➤ Keep your shoulders relaxed, your abs tight, and your sternum lifted.

tree pose

This exercise challenges your sense of balance and opens your hips.

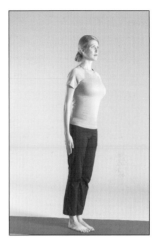

STARTING POSITION

Begin in Mountain Pose—stand straight, legs and toes together, heels slightly apart. Inhale and pull your abs toward your spine.

1. Place your palms together in front of your chest and lift one foot so that the sole of your foot is flat against your ankle, knee pointing to the side.

2. Keeping your palms together, lift your arms straight overhead and slide your working leg up so that the sole of your foot is flat against your thigh.

3. Hold for 5 breaths.

Repeat with other leg.

tip **from your personal trainer**

TO MODIFY:
Place the sole of your foot on your calf instead of your thigh. Use your hand to pull your leg up as high as you can.

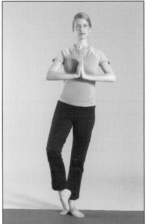

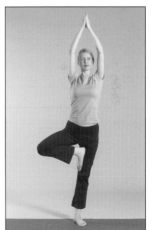

side forward bend

This exercise stretches your hamstrings, opens your hips, and warms up your spine.

STARTING POSITION

Stand with your legs apart, feet just wider than your shoulders. Place your hands on your hips.

1. Turn your right foot out to a 90-degree angle.

2. Rotate your hips toward your out-turned foot and bend forward, keeping your spine straight.

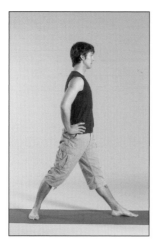 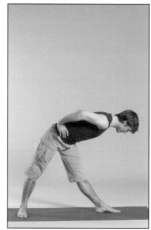

3. Roll your spine down as you relax your head to your knee.

4. Hold for 5 breaths.

HOT BOD FUSION

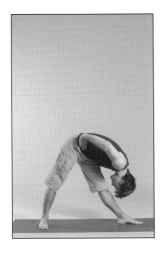
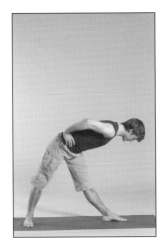
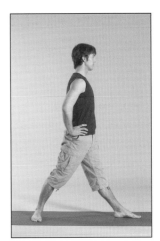

5. Roll your spine back up and rotate your hips back to Starting Position.

Repeat on other side.

tip **from your personal trainer**

TO INTENSIFY:
Place your arms behind your back, palms together.

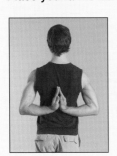
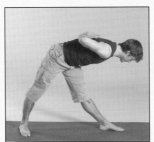
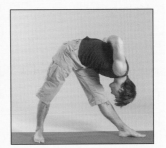

BALANCE CHALLENGERS

triangle pose moving

This classic movement stretches your hamstrings and your spine.

STARTING POSITION

Stand with your legs apart, feet wider than your shoulders.
Spread your arms out to your sides at shoulder height like wings.

1. Turn your left foot out to a 90-degree angle. Turn your right foot slightly in.

2. Shift the left side of your body over your left leg as you stretch out and down until you can touch your left hand to the mat by your outturned foot. Hold for 5 breaths.

3. Rotate your torso to face the mat and bring your right arm down to touch the mat.

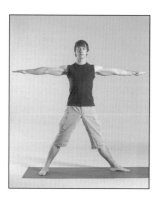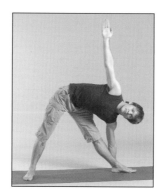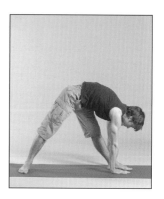

4. Keeping your right arm on the mat, rotate even further to face back as you lift your left arm up and toward the ceiling. Hold for 5 breaths.

5. Rotate back down and return your left arm to the mat.

6. Keeping your left arm on the mat, rotate even further as you lift your right arm up and toward the ceiling. Keep your pelvis square to the floor. Hold for 5 breaths.

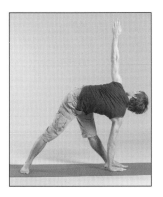 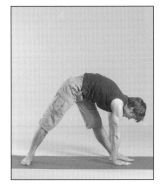 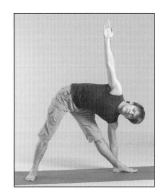

7. Return to Starting Position.

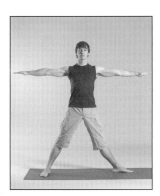

Repeat entire sequence on other side.

 tip

from your personal trainer

Keep your torso long and straight as you bend down.

TO MODIFY:
Place your hand on your shin instead of reaching all the way to the mat. Or bend your knee slightly.

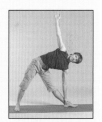

TO INTENSIFY:
Look toward your lifted hand.

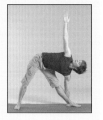

BALANCE CHALLENGERS

warrior I to warrior II to standing T

These movements flow from one into another, challenging your control and balance.

STARTING POSITION

Stand with your legs apart, feet wider than your shoulders. Spread your arms out to your sides at shoulder height with your palms facing down.

WARRIOR I

1. Rotate your torso and hips to the right and move your left leg to the side so that your foot is just inside your left hand. Point your toes out and bend your knee at a 90-degree angle. Your right leg should be straight.

2. As you lift up through your torso and extend your spine, raise your arms overhead and bring your palms together. Look up at your hands. Hold for 5 breaths.

3. Rotate back to center as you return your arms and legs to Starting Position.

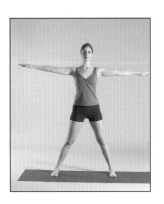 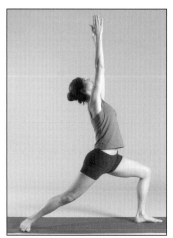 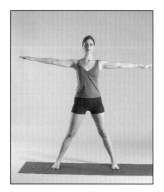

WARRIOR II

1. Move your left leg to the side so that your foot is just inside your left hand. Point your toes out and bend your knee at a 90-degree angle. Your right leg should be straight.

2. Turn your head to look over your left arm as you stretch both arms out as long as you can. Hold for 5 breaths.

3. Turn your head back to center as you return your legs to Starting Position.

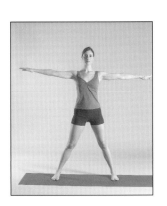 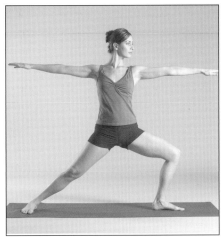 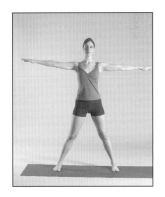

STANDING T

1. Rotate your torso to the left and turn your left foot out to the side.

2. Bend your left leg and flex forward at the hips. Lean toward your left leg and lift your right leg horizontal to the floor, while simultaneously straightening your left leg.

BALANCE CHALLENGERS ▬

warrior I to warrior II to standing T *(continued)*

3. Balance on your left leg and hold for 5 breaths.

4. Lower your leg and return to Starting Position.

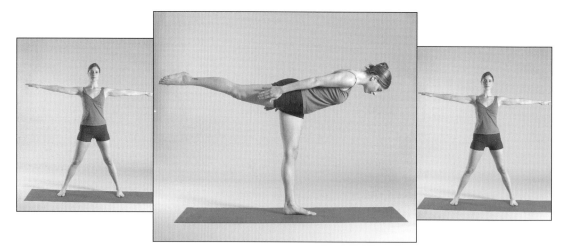

Repeat entire sequence on other side.

 tip **from your personal trainer**

➤ In Warrior I and Warrior II, be careful not to let your knee bend past your foot.
Position your bent knee directly over your ankle.

➤ In Warrior II, keep your hips facing forward.

➤ In Standing T, try to have your head, torso, and lifted leg parallel to the floor.

TO MODIFY:
In Standing T, hold the back of a chair or a table for balance.

side angle pose

This exercise is a side stretch that improves spinal flexibility and posture.

STARTING POSITION

Stand with your legs apart, just wider than your shoulders. Turn your left foot out and place your hands on your hips.

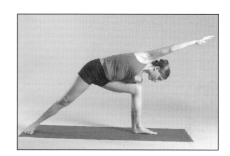

1. Bend your left knee and place your left hand on the mat next to the outside of your foot.

2. Stretch your right arm out long over your head. Hold for 5 breaths.

3. Return to Starting Position.

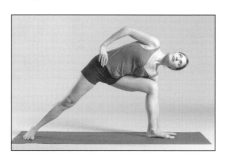

Repeat entire sequence with other leg.

 from your personal trainer

TO MODIFY:
Do not stretch your arm out over your head. Leave it on your hip.

TO INTENSIFY:
Look up toward your outstretched arm as you hold the pose.

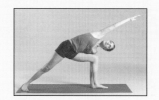

BALANCE CHALLENGERS ▬

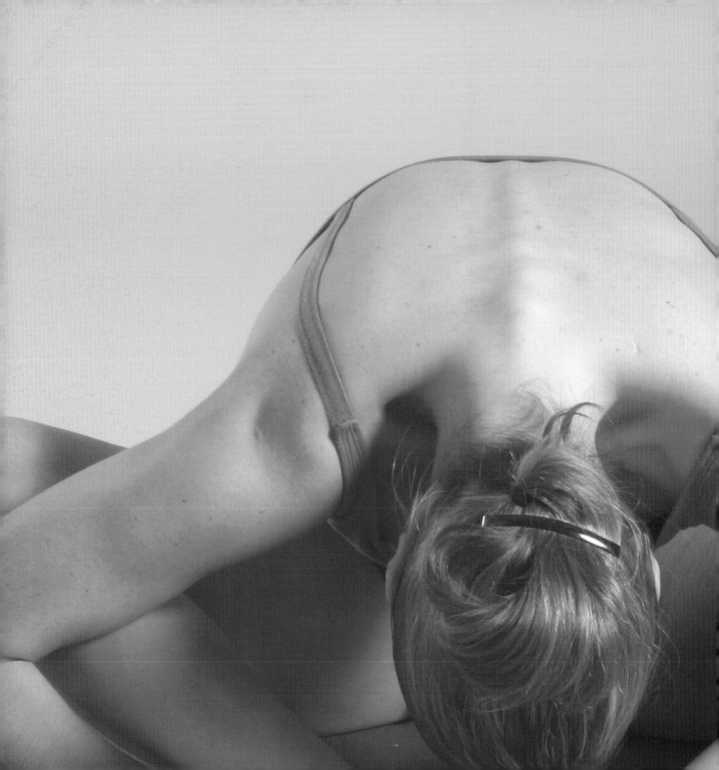

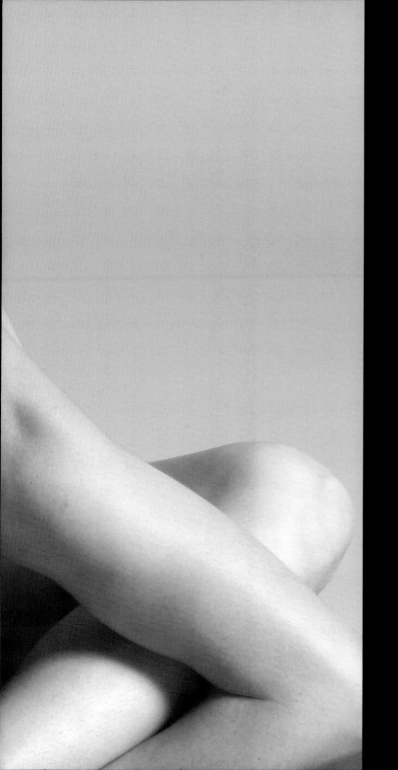

phase four

THE FINAL STRETCH

(Five-minute cool-down)

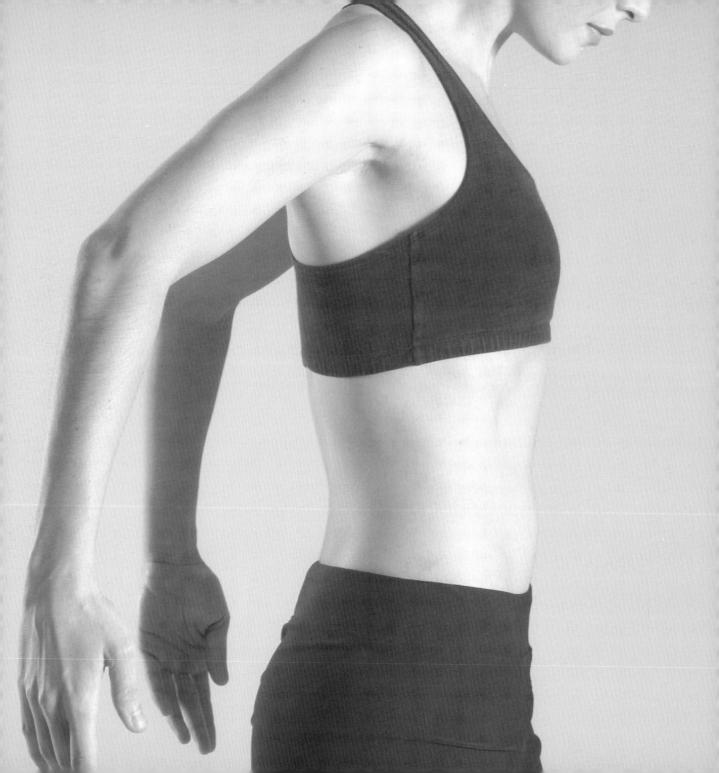

eleven

THE
COOL-DOWN

PILATES, BALLET,
AND YOGA

*T*HIS FIVE-MINUTE stretch melds movements from Pilates, ballet, and yoga. Stretching after you complete your workout is important for releasing any leftover tension and helping you wind down.

straddle stretch

There's a lot of punch packed into this simple stretch. You're working your hamstrings, adductors, lower back, and obliques.

STARTING POSITION

Sit upright, legs open in a V as wide as is comfortable. Rest your arms on your legs.

1. Reach up and out of your hip socket and stretch to the side as you bring one arm up and over. Your other arm is stretched long on your leg. Hold for 4 slow breaths.

2. Rotate your torso in the direction of your stretch and place both hands on either side of your leg. Hold for 4 slow breaths.

3. Keeping your torso rotated sideways, roll back up to vertical position.

4. Rotate your torso even more toward the back of the room and hold for 4 slow breaths.

5. Rotate your torso slowly back to center.

Repeat on your other side.
Repeat the entire sequence twice.

146

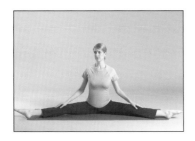
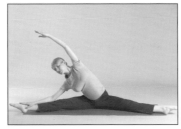
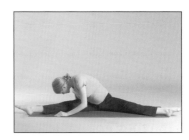

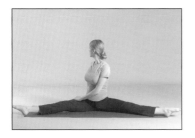
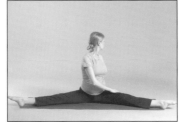
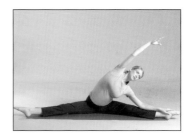

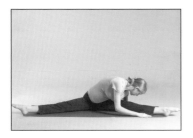
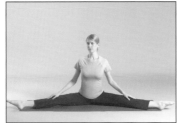
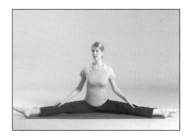

tip **from your personal trainer**

➤ Keep your knees facing up.
➤ Slide your shoulders down and
  back.

THE COOL-DOWN ▬

butterfly, forehead rest

Use this movement to relax and stretch your adductors and to stretch your hip joints.

STARTING POSITION

Sit upright with your knees bent and the soles of your feet together, heels about two feet away from your body. Rest your hands on your ankles.

1. Lean forward, aiming your forehead for the soles of your feet.

2. Relax and breathe naturally for 4 or more full breaths.

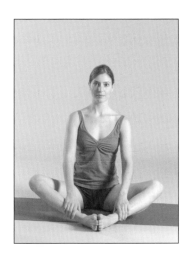

tip **from your personal trainer**

TO MODIFY:
Place your hands on your knees or at your sides.

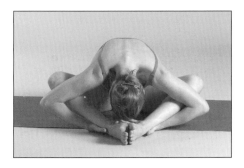

148

forward bend

This restful pose will stretch your back and hamstrings.

STARTING POSITION

Sit upright with your legs together and stretched out in front of you.

1. Lean your upper body over your legs. Place your palms flat at your sides or reaching for your feet.

2. Breathe naturally and hold this resting position for 4 or more full breaths.

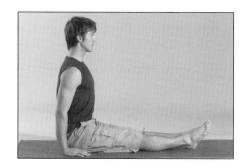

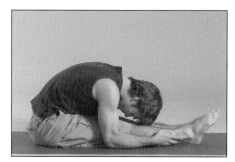

 tip

from your personal trainer

Sit on a pillow or bolster if you feel any lower back discomfort.

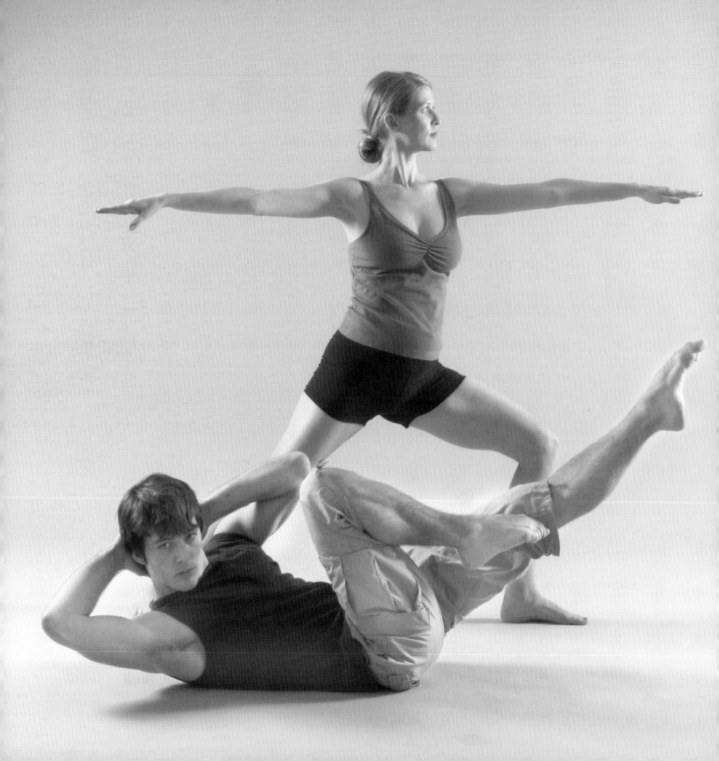

twelve

PUTTING IT ALL TOGETHER

HOW TO CREATE YOUR OWN WORKOUT

*t*HE EXERCISE FORMAT that we designed for *Hot Bod Fusion* allows you to customize your workout and change it from day to day—all year long. All the exercises will give you an effective workout, so feel free to mix and match them as you wish.

The following handy reference charts will help get you started. You can use them to keep track of which chapters you've used, how far you've come, and to monitor your progress. We suggest you make photocopies of these blank charts so that once you've filled one in, you'll have another one ready for your next sequence. In this way, you can create a different workout each day and continue on with this program indefinitely.

Fill in the blanks with your choice of one chapter from Phase Two and one chapter from Phase Three. Remember to always include the warm-up in Chapter 2 and the cool-down in Chapter 11. On cardio days, we suggest you do a minimum of twenty minutes of any type of cardiovascular activity.

You can choose between a four-week sequence and a five-week sequence that utilizes the optional exercise circle.

Four-Week Sequence

	MONDAY	TUESDAY	WEDNESDAY	THURSDAY	FRIDAY
WEEK 1		Cardio		Cardio	
WEEK 2	Cardio		Cardio		Cardio
WEEK 3		Cardio		Cardio	
WEEK 4	Cardio		Cardio		Cardio

Five-Week Sequence

(Using the Exercise Circle)

	MONDAY	TUESDAY	WEDNESDAY	THURSDAY	FRIDAY
WEEK 1		Cardio		Cardio	
WEEK 2		Cardio		Cardio	
WEEK 3		Cardio		Cardio	
WEEK 4		Cardio		Cardio	
WEEK 5		Cardio		Cardio	

HOW TO USE THE SAMPLE SEQUENCES

If you're not ready to create your own workout yet, just use the two sample sequence guides we've provided below. Don't forget to complete Chapter 2 (The Warm-Up) and Chapter 11 (The Cool-Down) in addition to the two chapters listed for each day in the chart. Make sure to do the exercises in sequential order to avoid repeating routines.

Sample Four-Week Sequence

	MONDAY	TUESDAY	WEDNESDAY	THURSDAY	FRIDAY
WEEK 1	Ch. 3, 7	Cardio	Ch. 6, 9	Cardio	Ch. 5, 7
WEEK 2	Cardio	Ch. 6, 10	Cardio	Ch. 3, 9	Cardio
WEEK 3	Ch. 5, 10	Cardio	Ch. 3, 10	Cardio	Ch. 6, 7
WEEK 4	Cardio	Ch. 5, 9	Cardio	You Choose!	Cardio

Sample Five-Week Sequence

(Using the Exercise Circle)

	MONDAY	TUESDAY	WEDNESDAY	THURSDAY	FRIDAY
WEEK 1	Ch. 3, 8	Cardio	Ch. 6, 9	Cardio	Ch. 5, 8
WEEK 2	Ch. 3, 9	Cardio	Ch. 4, 10	Cardio	Ch. 5, 9
WEEK 3	Ch. 6, 10	Cardio	Ch. 4, 7	Cardio	Ch. 3, 10
WEEK 4	Ch. 6, 7	Cardio	Ch. 5, 10	Cardio	Ch. 4, 8
WEEK 5	Ch. 5, 7	Cardio	Ch. 6, 8	Cardio	Ch. 4, 9

The authors would like to thank:

Dave Robie, from Big Score Productions, for believing in this project and working hard to find the right publisher.

Sue McCloskey, our editor at Marlowe & Company, for her editorial guidance and insightful suggestions.

Steve Ladner for his expert photographs and creativity.

The fitness models, Jennifer Capriccio and Terry Dean Bartlett, for their professionalism at the photo shoot.

acknowledgments